BMAT Practice Papers

Volume One

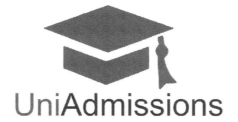

UniAdmissions

Copyright © 2018 *UniAdmissions*. All rights reserved.

ISBN 978-1-912557-21-9

Published by *RAR Medical Services Limited*
www.uniadmissions.co.uk
info@uniadmissions.co.uk
Tel: 0208 068 0438

BMAT Practice Papers

4 Full Papers & Solutions

Matthew Williams
Rohan Agarwal

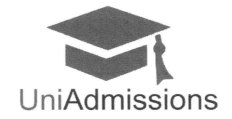

UniAdmissions

About the Authors

Matthew is **Resources Editor** at *UniAdmissions* and a final year medical student at St Catherine's College, Oxford. As the first student from Barry Comprehensive School in South Wales to receive a place on the Oxford medicine course he embraced all aspects of university life, both social and academic. Matt Scored in the **top 5% for his UKCAT and BMAT** to secure his offer at the University of Oxford.

Matthew has worked with UniAdmissions since 2014 – tutoring several applicants successfully into Oxbridge and Russell group universities. His work has been published in international scientific journals and he has presented his research at conferences across the globe. In his spare time, Matt enjoys playing rugby and golf.

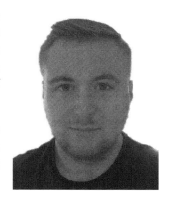

Rohan is the **Director of Operations** at *UniAdmissions* and is responsible for its technical and commercial arms. He graduated from Gonville and Caius College, Cambridge and is a fully qualified doctor. Over the last five years, he has tutored hundreds of successful Oxbridge and Medical applicants. He has also authored twenty books on admissions tests and interviews.

Rohan has taught physiology to undergraduate medical students and interviewed medical school applicants for Cambridge. He has published research on bone physiology and writes education articles for the Independent and Huffington Post. In his spare time, Rohan enjoys playing the piano and table tennis.

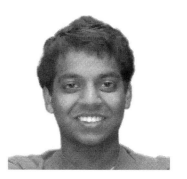

INTRODUCTION

The Basics

The BioMedical Admissions Test (BMAT) is the 2-hour written aptitude exam taken by students applying for Medicine, Biomedical Sciences, Dentistry, and Veterinary Medicine courses at the most competitive universities.

It is a highly time pressured exam that forces you to apply GCSE and A-level knowledge in ways you have never thought about before. In this respect simply remembering solutions taught in class or from past papers is not enough.

However, fear not, despite what people say, you can actually prepare for the BMAT! With a little practice you can train your brain to manipulate and apply learnt methodologies to novel problems with ease. The best way to do this is through exposure to as many past/specimen papers as you can.

Preparing for the BMAT

Before going any further, it's important that you understand the optimal way to prepare for the BMAT. Rather than jumping straight into doing mock papers, it's essential that you start by understanding the components and the theory behind the BMAT by using an BMAT textbook. Once you've finished the non-timed practice questions, you can progress to past BMAT papers. These are freely available online at **www.uniadmissions.co.uk/bmat-past-papers** and serve as excellent practice. You're strongly advised to use these in combination with the *BMAT Past Worked Solutions* Book so that you can improve your weaknesses. Finally, once you've exhausted past papers, move onto the mock papers in this book.

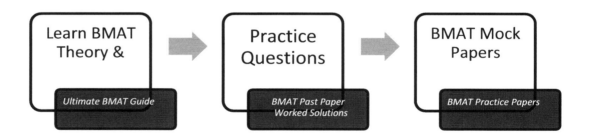

Already seen them all?

So, you've run out of past papers? Well hopefully that is where this book comes in. It contains eight unique mock papers; each compiled by expert BMAT tuors at *UniAdmissions* who scored in the top 10% nationally.

Having successfully gained a place on their course of choice, our tutors are intimately familiar with the BMAT and its associated admission procedures. So, the novel questions presented to you here are of the correct style and difficulty to continue your revision and stretch you to meet the demands of the BMAT.

General Advice

Start Early

It is much easier to prepare if you practice little and often. Start your preparation well in advance; ideally 10 weeks but at the latest within a month. This way you will have plenty of time to complete as many papers as you wish to feel comfortable and won't have to panic and cram just before the test, which is a much less effective and more stressful way to learn. In general, an early start will give you the opportunity to identify the complex issues and work at your own pace.

Prioritise

Some questions in sections can be long and complex – and given the intense time pressure you need to know your limits. It is essential that you don't get stuck with very difficult questions. If a question looks particularly long or complex, mark it for review and move on. You don't want to be caught 5 questions short at the end just because you took more than 3 minutes in answering a challenging multi-step question. If a question is taking too long, choose a sensible answer and move on. Remember that each question carries equal weighting and therefore, you should adjust your timing in accordingly. With practice and discipline, you can get very good at this and learn to maximise your efficiency.

Positive Marking

There are no penalties for incorrect answers; you will gain one for each right answer and will not get one for each wrong or unanswered one. This provides you with the luxury that you can always guess should you absolutely be not able to figure out the right answer for a question or run behind time. Since each question provides you with 4 to 6 possible answers, you have a 16-25% chance of guessing correctly. Therefore, if you aren't sure (and are running short of time), then make an educated guess and move on. Before 'guessing' you should try to eliminate a couple of answers to increase your chances of getting the question correct. For example, if a question has 5 options and you manage to eliminate 2 options- your chances of getting the question increase from 20% to 33%!

Avoid losing easy marks on other questions because of poor exam technique. Similarly, if you have failed to finish the exam, take the last 10 seconds to guess the remaining questions to at least give yourself a chance of getting them right.

Practice

This is the best way of familiarising yourself with the style of questions and the timing for this section. Although the exam will essentially only test GCSE level knowledge, you are unlikely to be familiar with the style of questions in all sections when you first encounter them. Therefore, you want to be comfortable at using this before you sit the test.

Practising questions will put you at ease and make you more comfortable with the exam. The more comfortable you are, the less you will panic on the test day and the more likely you are to score highly. Initially, work through the questions at your own pace, and spend time carefully reading the questions and looking at any additional data. When it becomes closer to the test, **make sure you practice the questions under exam conditions**.

Past Papers

Official past papers and answers from 2003 onwards are freely available online on our website at **www.uniadmissions.co.uk/bmat-past-papers**. Keep in mind that the specification was changed in 2009 so some things asked in earlier papers may not be representative of the content that is currently examinable in the BMAT. In general, **it is worth doing at least all the papers from 2009 onwards**. Time permitting; you can work backwards from 2009 although there is little point doing the section 3 essays pre-2009 as they are significantly different to the current style of essays.

You will undoubtedly get stuck when doing some past paper questions – they are designed to be tricky and the answer schemes don't offer any explanations. Thus, **you're highly advised to acquire a copy of *BMAT Past Paper Worked Solutions*** – a free ebook is available online (see the back of this book for more details).

Repeat Questions

When checking through answers, pay particular attention to questions you have got wrong. If there is a worked answer, look through that carefully until you feel confident that you understand the reasoning, and then repeat the question without help to check that you can do it. If only the answer is given, have another look at the question and try to work out why that answer is correct. This is the best way to learn from your mistakes, and means you are less likely to make similar mistakes when it comes to the test. The same applies for questions which you were unsure of and made an educated guess which was correct, even if you got it right. When working through this book, **make sure you highlight any questions you are unsure of**, this means you know to spend more time looking over them once marked.

No Calculators

You aren't permitted to use calculators in the exam – thus, it is essential that you have strong numerical skills. For instance, you should be able to rapidly convert between percentages, decimals and fractions. You will seldom get questions that would require calculators, but you would be expected to be able to arrive at a sensible estimate. Consider for example:

Estimate 3.962 x 2.322;

3.962 is approximately 4 and 2.323 is approximately 2.33 = 7/3.

Thus,
$$3.962 \times 2.322 \approx 4 \times \frac{7}{3} = \frac{28}{3} = 9.33$$

Since you will rarely be asked to perform difficult calculations, you can use this as a signpost of if you are tackling a question correctly. For example, when solving a physics question, you end up having to divide 8,079 by 357- this should raise alarm bells as calculations in the BMAT are rarely this difficult.

> *Top tip!* In general, students tend to improve the fastest in section 2 and slowest in section 1; section 3 usually falls somewhere in the middle. Thus, if you have very little time left, it's best to prioritise section 2.

A word on timing...

"If you had all day to do your exam, you would get 100%. But you don't."
Whilst this isn't completely true, it illustrates a very important point. Once you've practiced and know how to answer the questions, the clock is your biggest enemy. This seemingly obvious statement has one very important consequence. **The way to improve your score is to improve your speed.** There is no magic bullet. But there are a great number of techniques that, with practice, will give you significant time gains, allowing you to answer more questions and score more marks.

Timing is tight throughout – **mastering timing is the first key to success**. Some candidates choose to work as quickly as possible to save up time at the end to check back, but this is generally not the best way to do it. Often questions can have a lot of information in them – each time you start answering a question it takes time to get familiar with the instructions and information. By splitting the question into two sessions (the first run-through and the return-to-check) you double the amount of time you spend on familiarising yourself with the data, as you have to do it twice instead of only once. This costs valuable time. In addition, candidates who do check back may spend 2–3 minutes doing so and yet not make any actual changes. Whilst this can be reassuring, it is a false reassurance as it is unlikely to have a significant effect on your actual score. Therefore, it is usually best to pace yourself very steadily, aiming to spend the same amount of time on each question and finish the final question in a section just as time runs out. This reduces the time spent on re-familiarising with questions and maximises the time spent on the first attempt, gaining more marks.

It is essential that you don't get stuck with the hardest questions – no doubt there will be some. In the time spent answering only one of these you may miss out on answering three easier questions. If a question is taking too long, choose a sensible answer and move on. Never see this as giving up or in any way failing, rather it is the smart way to approach a test with a tight time limit. With practice and discipline, you can get very good at this and learn to maximise your efficiency. It is not about being a hero and aiming for full marks – this is almost impossible and very much unnecessary (even Oxbridge will regard any score higher than 7 as exceptional). It is about maximising your efficiency and gaining the maximum possible number of marks within the time you have.

Use the Options:

Some questions may try to overload you with information. When presented with large tables and data, it's essential you look at the answer options so you can focus your mind. This can allow you to reach the correct answer a lot more quickly. Consider the example below:

The table below shows the results of a study investigating antibiotic resistance in staphylococcus populations. A single staphylococcus bacterium is chosen at random from a similar population. Resistance to any one antibiotic is independent of resistance to others.

Calculate the probability that the bacterium selected will be resistant to all four drugs.

A   1 in 10^6
B   1 in 10^{12}
C   1 in 10^{20}
D   1 in 10^{25}
E   1 in 10^{30}
F   1 in 10^{35}

Antibiotic	Number of Bacteria tested	Number of Resistant Bacteria
Benzyl-penicillin	10^{11}	98
Chloramphenicol	10^9	1200
Metronidazole	10^8	256
Erythromycin	10^5	2

Looking at the options first makes it obvious that there is **no need to calculate exact values**- only in powers of 10. This makes your life a lot easier. If you hadn't noticed this, you might have spent well over 90 seconds trying to calculate the exact value when it wasn't even being asked for.

In other cases, you may actually be able to use the options to arrive at the solution quicker than if you had tried to solve the question as you normally would. Consider the example below:

A region is defined by the two inequalities: $x - y^2 > 1 \ and \ xy > 1$. Which of the following points is in the defined region?

A. (10,3)
B. (10,2)
C. (-10,3)
D. (-10,2)
E. (-10,-3)

Whilst it's possible to solve this question both algebraically or graphically by manipulating the identities, by far **the quickest way is to actually use the options**. Note that options C, D and E violate the second inequality, narrowing down to answer to either A or B. For A: $10 - 3^2 = 1$ and thus this point is on the boundary of the defined region and not actually in the region. Thus the answer is B (as 10-4 = 6 > 1.)

In general, it pays dividends to look at the options briefly and see if they can be help you arrive at the question more quickly. Get into this habit early – it may feel unnatural at first but it's guaranteed to save you time in the long run.

Keywords

If you're stuck on a question; pay particular attention to the options that contain key modifiers like "**always**", "**only**", "**all**" as examiners like using them to test if there are any gaps in your knowledge. E.g. the statement "arteries carry oxygenated blood" would normally be true; "All arteries carry oxygenated blood" would be false because the pulmonary artery carries deoxygenated blood.

Manage your Time:

It is highly likely that you will be juggling your revision alongside your normal school studies. Whilst it is tempting to put your A-levels on the back burner falling behind in your school subjects is not a good idea, don't forget that to meet the conditions of your offer should you get one you will need at least one A*. So, time management is key!

Make sure you set aside a dedicated 90 minutes (and much more closer to the exam) to commit to your revision each day. The key here is not to sacrifice too many of your extracurricular activities, everybody needs some down time, but instead to be efficient. Take a look at our list of top tips for increasing revision efficiency below:

1. Create a comfortable work station
2. Declutter and stay tidy
3. Treat yourself to some nice stationery
4. See if music works for you → if not, find somewhere peaceful and quiet to work
5. Turn off your mobile or at least put it into silent mode
6. Silence social media alerts
7. Keep the TV off and out of sight
8. Stay organised with to do lists and revision timetables – more importantly, stick to them!
9. Keep to your set study times and don't bite off more than you can chew
10. Study while you're commuting
11. Adopt a positive mental attitude
12. Get into a routine
13. Consider forming a study group to focus on the harder exam concepts
14. Plan rest and reward days into your timetable – these are excellent incentive for you to stay on track with your study plans!

Keep Fit & Eat Well:

'A car won't work if you fill it with the wrong fuel' - your body is exactly the same. You cannot hope to perform unless you remain fit and well. The best way to do this is not underestimate the importance of healthy eating. Beige, starchy foods will make you sluggish; instead start the day with a hearty breakfast like porridge. Aim for the recommended 'five a day' intake of fruit/veg and stock up on the oily fish or blueberries – the so called "super foods".

When hitting the books, it's essential to keep your brain hydrated. If you get dehydrated you'll find yourself lethargic and possibly developing a headache, neither of which will do any favours for your revision. Invest in a good water bottle that you know the total volume of and keep sipping through the day. Don't forget that the amount of water you should be aiming to drink varies depending on your mass, so calculate your own personal recommended intake as follows: 30 ml per kg per day.

It is well known that exercise boosts your wellbeing and instils a sense of discipline. All of which will reflect well in your revision. It's well worth devoting half an hour a day to some exercise, get your heart rate up, break a sweat, and get those endorphins flowing.

Sleep

It's no secret that when revising you need to keep well rested. Don't be tempted to stay up late revising as sleep actually plays an important part in consolidating long term memory. Instead aim for a minimum of 7 hours good sleep each night, in a dark room without any glow from electronic appliances. Install flux (https://justgetflux.com) on your laptop to prevent your computer from disrupting your circadian rhythm. Aim to go to bed the same time each night and no hitting snooze on the alarm clock in the morning!

Revision Timetable

Still struggling to get organised? Then try filling in the example revision timetable below, remember to factor in enough time for short breaks, and stick to it! Remember to schedule in several breaks throughout the day and actually use them to do something you enjoy e.g. TV, reading, YouTube etc.

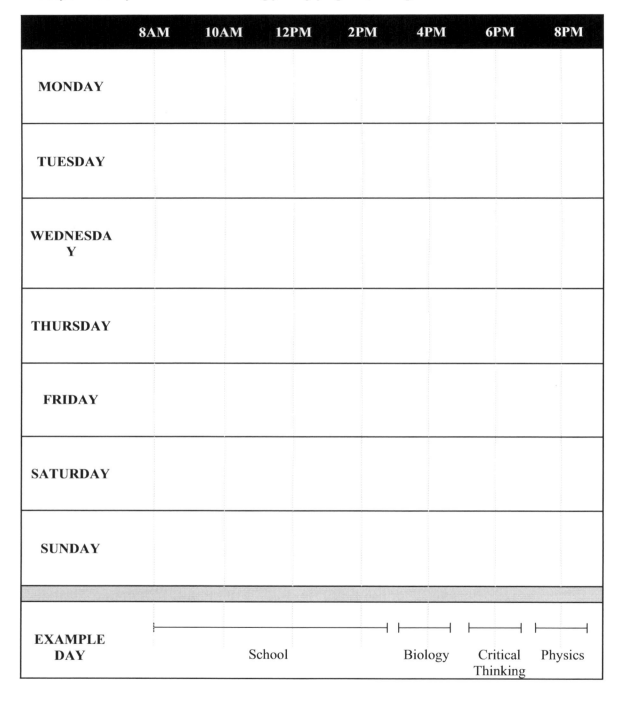

	8AM	10AM	12PM	2PM	4PM	6PM	8PM
MONDAY							
TUESDAY							
WEDNESDAY							
THURSDAY							
FRIDAY							
SATURDAY							
SUNDAY							
EXAMPLE DAY	School				Biology	Critical Thinking	Physics

Top tip! Ensure that you take a watch that can show you the time in seconds into the exam. This will allow you have a much more accurate idea of the time you're spending on a question. In general, if you've spent >150 seconds on a section 1 question or >90 seconds on a section 2 questions – move on regardless of how close you think you are to solving it.

Getting the most out of Mock Papers

Mock exams can prove invaluable if tackled correctly. Not only do they encourage you to start revision earlier, they also allow you to **practice and perfect your revision technique**. They are often the best way of improving your knowledge base or reinforcing what you have learnt. Probably the best reason for attempting mock papers is to familiarise yourself with the exam conditions of the BMAT as they are particularly tough.

Start Revision Earlier

Thirty five percent of students agree that they procrastinate to a degree that is detrimental to their exam performance. This is partly explained by the fact that they often seem a long way in the future. In the scientific literature this is well recognised, Dr. Piers Steel, an expert on the field of motivation states that *'the further away an event is, the less impact it has on your decisions'*.

Mock exams are therefore a way of giving you a target to work towards and motivate you in the run up to the real thing – every time you do one treat it as the real deal! If you do well then it's a reassuring sign; if you do poorly then it will motivate you to work harder (and earlier!).

Practice and perfect revision techniques

In case you haven't realised already, revision is a skill all to itself, and can take some time to learn. For example, the most common revision techniques including **highlighting and/or re-reading are quite ineffective** ways of committing things to memory. Unless you are thinking critically about something you are much less likely to remember it or indeed understand it.

Mock exams, therefore allow you to test your revision strategies as you go along. Try spacing out your revision sessions so you have time to forget what you have learnt in-between. This may sound counterintuitive but the second time you remember it for longer. Try teaching another student what you have learnt, this forces you to structure the information in a logical way that may aid memory. Always try to question what you have learnt and appraise its validity. Not only does this aid memory but it is also a useful skill for BMAT section 3, Oxbridge interview, and beyond.

Improve your knowledge

The act of applying what you have learnt reinforces that piece of knowledge. A question may ask you to think about a relatively basic concept in a novel way (not cited in textbooks), and so deepen your understanding. Exams rarely test word for word what is in the syllabus, so when running through mock papers try to understand how the basic facts are applied and tested in the exam. As you go through the mocks or past papers take note of your performance and see if you consistently under-perform in specific areas, thus highlighting areas for future study.

Get familiar with exam conditions

Pressure can cause all sorts of trouble for even the most brilliant students. The BMAT is a particularly time pressured exam with high stakes – your future (without exaggerating) does depend on your result to a great extent. The real key to the BMAT is overcoming this pressure and remaining calm to allow you to think efficiently.

Mock exams are therefore an excellent opportunity to devise and perfect your own exam techniques to beat the pressure and meet the demands of the exam. **Don't treat mock exams like practice questions – it's imperative you do them under time conditions.**

> *Remember!* It's better that you make all the mistakes you possibly can now in mock papers and then learn from them so as not to repeat them in the real exam.

Things to have done before using this book

Do the ground work

➤ Read in detail: the background, methods, and aims of the BMAT as well logistical considerations such as how to take the BMAT in practice. A good place to start is a BMAT textbook like *The Ultimate BMAT Guide* (flick to the back to get a free copy!) which covers all the groundwork but it's also worth looking through the official BMAT site (www.admissionstesting.org/bmat).

➤ It is generally a good idea to start re-capping all your GCSE maths and science.

➤ Practice substituting formulas together to reach a more useful one expressing known variables e.g. $P = IV$ and $V = IR$ can be combined to give $P = V^2/R$ and $P = I^2R$. Remember that calculators are not permitted in the exam, so get comfortable doing more complex long addition, multiplication, division, and subtraction.

➤ Get comfortable rapidly converting between percentages, decimals, and fractions.

➤ Practice developing logical arguments and structuring essays with an obvious introduction, main body, and ending.

➤ These are all things which are easiest to do alongside your revision for exams before the summer break. Not only gaining a head start on your BMAT revision but also complimenting your year 12 studies well.

➤ Discuss scientific problems with others - propose experiments and state what you think the result would be. Be ready to defend your argument. This will rapidly build your scientific understanding for section 2 but also prepare you well for an oxbridge interview.

➤ Read through the BMAT syllabus before you start tackling whole papers. This is absolutely essential. It contains several stated formulae, constants, and facts that you are expected to apply - or may just be an answer in their own right. Familiarising yourself with the syllabus is also a quick way of teaching yourself the additional information other exam boards may learn which you do not. Sifting through the whole BMAT syllabus is a time-consuming process so we have done it for you. **Be sure to flick through the syllabus checklist** later on, which also doubles up as a great revision aid for the night before!

Ease in gently

With the ground work laid, there's still no point in adopting exam conditions straight away. Instead invest in a beginner's guide to the BMAT, which will not only describe in detail the background and theory of the exam, but take you through section by section what is expected. *The Ultimate BMAT Guide: 800 Practice Questions* is the most popular BMAT textbook – you can get a free copy by flicking to the back of this book.

When you are ready to move on to past papers, take your time and puzzle your way through all the questions. Really try to understand solutions. A past paper question won't be repeated in your real exam, so don't rote learn methods or facts. Instead, focus on applying prior knowledge to formulate your own approach.

If you're really struggling and have to take a sneak peek at the answers, then practice thinking of alternative solutions, or arguments for essays. It is unlikely that your answer will be more elegant or succinct than the model answer, but it is still a good task for encouraging creativity with your thinking. Get used to thinking outside the box!

Accelerate and Intensify

Start adopting exam conditions after you've done two past papers. Don't forget that **it's the time pressure that makes the BMAT hard** – if you had as long as you wanted to sit the exam you would probably get 100%. If you're struggling to find comprehensive answers to past papers then *BMAT Past Papers Worked Solutions* contains detailed explained answers to every BMAT past paper question and essay (flick to the back to get a free copy).

Doing all the past papers from 2009 – present is a good target for your revision. Note that the BMAT syllabus changed in 2009 so questions before this date may no longer be relevant. In any case, choose a paper and proceed with strict exam conditions. Take a short break and then mark your answers before reviewing your progress. For revision purposes, as you go along, keep track of those questions that you guess – these are equally as important to review as those you get wrong.

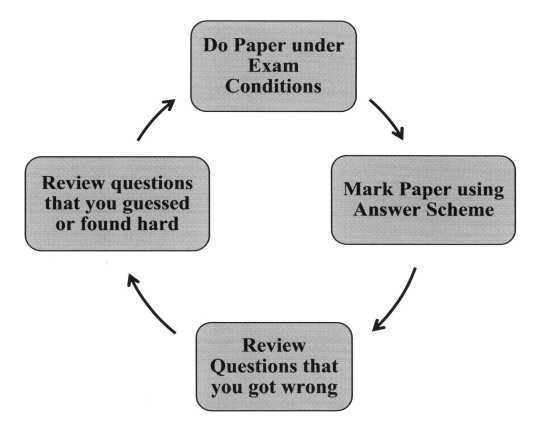

Once you've exhausted all the past papers, move on to tackling the unique mock papers in this book. In general, you should aim to complete one to two mock papers every night in the ten days preceding your exam.

Section 1: An Overview

What will you be tested on?	No. of Questions	Duration
Generic skills in problem solving, understanding arguments, and data analysis and inference.	35 MCQs	60 Minutes

This is the first section of the BMAT, comprising what most people describe as the classic IQ test style questions. Giving you one hour to answer 35 questions testing your ability to think critically, solve problems, and handle data. Breaking things down you realise that you are left with approximately 100 seconds per question. Remember though that this not only includes reasoning your answers, but also reading passages of text and/or analysing diagrams or graphs.

Not all the questions are of equal difficulty and so as you work through the past material it is certainly worth learning to recognise quickly which questions you need to skip to avoid getting bogged down. If it comes to it and you do not have enough time to go back to any skipped questions at the end, you always have a 20% chance of getting the answer correct with a guess!

Critical thinking questions

These types of question will generally present you with a passage of text or a methodology for an experiment and ask you to do one of three things: identify a conclusion, identify and assumption or flaw, or give an argument to either strengthen or weaken the statement.

The ability to filter through irrelevant material is essential with these questions as well as a solid grasp of the English language. Remember to only use the information given to you in your reasoning and never be too general with your conclusions – seek direct evidence in the information given. Critical thinking questions are definitely an example of when it is **best to read the question first**!

Problem solving questions

The problems in section 1 are often very wordy and complex, therefore it is often useful to turn the prose of the question into a series of equations. For example, being able to turn the sentence "Megan is half as tall as Elin" into "$2M = E$" should become second nature to you. Trial and error is not a method you should adopt for any questions in section 1 as it is far too time consuming.

As you are working through the preparation material try to get used to recognising which questions can be aided by drawing a quick diagram. This could apply to questions asking about timetables, orders, sequences, or spatial relationships. Remember it doesn't have to be pretty, merely help you organise your thoughts!

Data handling questions

These questions will undoubtedly require you to work with numbers, often calculating percentages or frequencies. Again, reading the question first can help you save time here, directing your attention to the relevant information in the passage. When analysing tables or graphs always check the following:

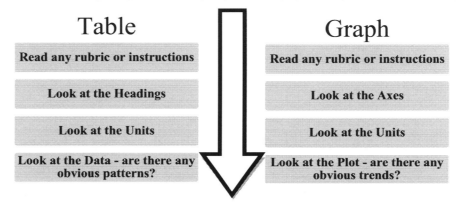

Table	Graph
Read any rubric or instructions	Read any rubric or instructions
Look at the Headings	Look at the Axes
Look at the Units	Look at the Units
Look at the Data - are there any obvious patterns?	Look at the Plot - are there any obvious trends?

Section 2: An Overview

What will you be tested on?	No. of Questions	Duration
The ability to apply scientific knowledge typically covered in school Science and Mathematics by 16	27 MCQs	30 Minutes

If you're short of time, then section 2 is where to focus. Undoubtedly the most time pressured section of the BMAT (requiring you to answer a question a minute) but also the section where candidates improve the fastest. Section 2 draws on your GCSE knowledge of biology, chemistry, physics, and maths.

It is important to remember that this is **GCSE knowledge taken from ALL exam boards**. So, you may find information that you are not familiar with if it was ignored by your exam board. To make sure you have a comprehensive knowledge of all the required material be sure to run through the section 2 revision checklists on the next few pages.

Biology

Generally, the biology questions require the least amount of time and are often where you can rely on making up lost time from harder questions. Most of biology questions rely on you being able to recall facts rather than interpret data or solve equations, so some good old-fashioned text book revision will prepare you well for these questions.

Chemistry

If you're taking the BMAT you will undoubtedly be studying chemistry at A-level as it is a requirement of all medical schools. Conceptually therefore, you should be in the clear, however, balancing complex equations or processing lengthy calculations can be time consuming.

Practicing with mock papers is essentially in combating this – really focus on extracting what the question is asking for as quickly as possible. In addition to the equations on the subsequent pages you must be comfortable with converting between litres, dm^3, cm^3, and mm^3 as well as using Avogadro's constant in calculations.

Physics

Physics is by far the most common subject that students drop moving on to AS-level, meaning these questions are the most poorly answered. There is a large variation in physics specifications between GCSE exam boards, so **before you do anything else read through the BMAT syllabus and commit all the stated equations and constants to memory** (helpfully highlighted in bold type on the revision checklist).

Physics questions will almost always require a two-step solution, normally forcing you to combine and re-arrange equations. All answers must be given in SI units which actually benefits you, by looking at the units you can often derive the equation – for example speed in m/s is calculated as distance(m) / time(s). It is also worth becoming fluent with the terminology for orders of magnitude in measurements (see right).

Factor	Text	Symbol
10^{12}	Tera	T
10^9	Giga	G
10^6	Mega	M
10^3	Kilo	k
10^2	Hecto	h
10^{-1}	Deci	d
10^{-2}	Centi	c
10^{-3}	Milli	m
10^{-6}	Micro	µ
10^{-9}	Nano	n
10^{-12}	Pico	p

Maths

Maths is the single most important component of section 2, a question topic in its own right but also applied in chemistry, physics, and section 1. Just remember to limit yourself to GCSE knowledge in the maths questions and don't overcomplicate things. As a bare minimum for preparation you should practice applying the quadratic formula, completing the square, and finding the difference between 2 squares.

Section 2: Revision Checklist

MATHS

Syllabus Point	What to Know
1. **Units**	Standard units of mass, length, time, money, and other measures Define compound units Change freely between related standard and compound units
2. **Number**	Order positive and negative integers, decimals, and fractions Understand and use $=, \neq, \leq, \geq, <, >$ Understand and use BIDMAS Define; factor, multiple, common factor, highest common factor, least common multiple, prime number, prime factor decomposition, square, positive and negative square root, cube and cube root Use index laws to simplify multiplication and division of powers Interpret, order and calculate with numbers written in standard index form Convert between fractions, decimals and percentages Understand and use direct and indirect proportion Apply the unitary method Use surds and π in exact calculations, simplify expressions that contain surds. Calculate upper and lower bounds to contextual problems Rounding to a given number of decimal places or significant figures
3. **Ratio and Proportion**	Use scale factors, diagrams, and maps Express a quantity as a fracation of another Express division of a quantity in two parts as a ratio Understand and use proportion Define percentage Work with percentages greater than 100% Solve problems using percentage change Appreciate why percentage can be used rather than a raw number
4. **Algebra**	Simplify rational expressions by cancelling or factorising and cancelling Set up quadratic equations and solve them by factorising Know the quadratic formula Set up and use equations to solve problems involving direct and indirect proportion Use linear expressions to describe the nth term of a sequence Use Cartesian coordinates in all four quadrants Equation of a straight line, $y=mx+c$, parallel lines have the same gradient Identify pairs of parallel and perpendicular lines Graphically solve simultaneous equations Recognise and interpret graphs of simple cubic functions, the reciprocal function, trigonometric functions and the exponential function $y=kx$ for integer values of x and simple positive values of k Draw transformations of $y=f(x)$ [$(y=af(x), y=f(a^x), y=f(x)+a, y=f(x-a)$ **only**] Deduce expressions to calculate the nth term in a sequence
5. **Geometry**	Recall and use properties of angle at a point, on a straight line, perpendicular lines and opposite angles at a vertex, and the sums of the interior and exterior angles of polygons Understand congruence and similarity Use Pythagoras' theorem in 2-D and 3-D Use the trigonometric ratios, between 0° and 180°, to solve problems in 2-D and 3-D Understand and construct geometrical proofs, including using circle theorems:

a. **the angle subtended at the circumference in a semicircle is a right angle**

b. **the tangent at any point on a circle is perpendicular to the radius at that point**

Describe and transform 2-D shapes using single or combined rotations, reflections, translations, or enlargements, including the use of vector notation

6.	**Measures**	Use conventional terms and notation
		Calculate perimeters and areas of shapes made from triangles, rectangles, and other shapes, find circumferences and areas of circles, including arcs and sectors
		Apply the standard circle theorems concerning angles, radii, tangents, and chords:
		• Angle subtended at the centre is twice the angle subtended at the circumference
		• Angle in a semicircle is 90°
		• Angles in the same segment are equal
		• Angle between a tangent and a chord (alternate segment theorem)
		• Angle between a radius and a tangent is 90°
		• Properties of cyclic quadrilaterals
		Calculate the volumes and surface areas of prisms, pyramids, spheres, cylinders, cones and solids made from cubes and cuboids (formulae given for the sphere and cone)
		Use vectors, including the sum of two vectors, algebraically and graphically
		Discuss the inaccuracies of measurements
		Understand and use three-figure bearings
7.	**Statistics**	Identify possible sources of bias in experimental methodology
		Discrete vs. continuous data
		Interpret cumulative frequency tables and graphs, box plots and histograms
		Define mean, median, mode, modal class, range, and inter-quartile range
		Interpret scatter diagrams and recognise correlation, drawing and using lines of best fit
		Compare sets of data by using statistical measures
8.	**Probability**	List all the outcomes for single and combined events
		Identify different mutually exclusive outcomes and know that the sum of the probabilities of all these outcomes is 1
		Construct and use Venn diagrams
		Know when to add or multiply two probabilities, and understand conditional probability
		Understand the use of tree diagrams to represent outcomes of combined events
		Compare experimental and theoretical probabilities
		Understand that if an experiment is repeated, the outcome may be different

BIOLOGY

Syllabus Point	What to Know
1. Cells	Differences in cellular structure and function between: -Animals: cell membrane, cytoplasm, nucleus, mitochondrion -Plants: cell membrane, cytoplasm, nucleus, cell wall, chloroplast, mitochondrion, vacuole -Bacteria: cell membrane, cytoplasm, cell wall, no true nucleus Multiple cells form tissues, several tissues form an organ
2. Movement Across Membranes	Difference between diffusion, osmosis, and active transport Role of cellular proteins Need for mitochondria in active transport
3. Cell Division & Sex	Define mitosis vs. meiosis Asexual vs. sexual reproduction Sex determination: females XX, males XY Calculate gender ratio
4. Inheritance	Role of nucleus in cell function Define genes, alleles, dominant, recessive, heterozygous, homozygous, phenotype, and genotype Use monohybrid crosses and family trees to calculate ratios/percentages Cystic fibrosis, polydactyly, and Huntington's
5. DNA	Chromosomes Structure of DNA Protein synthesis from DNA base triplets
6. Gene Technologies	Methods of experimental gene insertion Roles of stem cells: embryonic vs. adult
7. Variation	Natural selection: variation, differential survival based on adaptation, only those best adapted survive to reproduce Antibiotic resistance (MRSA) Genetic vs. environmental causes of variation Extinction occurs when organisms can't adapt quickly enough
8. Enzymes	Define biological catalyst Mechanism of action: lock and key vs. induced fit Effects of temperature and pH The role of amylase, protease, and lipase
9. Animal Physiology	Define and describe aerobic and anaerobic respiration Define homeostasis Negative vs. positive feedback Regulation of blood glucose, water, and temperature Function of white blood cells Hormones: travel in blood to target organs Structure (anatomy), organisation, and function of the: -Nervous system: sensory vs. motor vs. relay neurons, reflex arcs, synapses -Respiratory system: thorax, process of ventilation and gas exchange -Circulatory system: sinoatrial node, atrioventricular node, heart rate and ECGs, differences between arteries, veins, and capillaries, blood groups -Digestive system: digestive enzymes, pH -Kidney: the nephron, role in homeostasis
10. Ecosystems	Food chains, energy flow Pyramids of biomass Define niche Factors affecting population growth Carbon cycle: photosynthesis, respiration, combustion, decomposition Nitrogen cycle: bacteria, nitrification, decomposition, nitrogen fixation,

denitrification

CHEMISTRY

Syllabus Point	What to Know
1. Atomic Structure	Structure of the atom Relative masses and charges of protons, neutrons, and electrons Atomic vs. mass number, electron configurations Isotope definition Define A_r, calculate M_r Mass spectrometry
2. Periodic Table	Organisation of periods vs. groups and metals vs. non-metals Displacement reactions and reactivity, extraction of metals from their ores Position of the alkali metals, halogens, noble gases, and transition metals, relate position to electron configuration Reactivity increases down a metal group but decreases down a non-metal group Properties of transition metals Calculate A_r from isotopic mass and abundance.
3. Reactions & Equations	Conservation of matter Endothermic vs. exothermic Charges of common polyatomic cations (e.g. CO_3^{2-}) Formulate equations describing redox reactions Factors that affect the position of equilibrium in reversible reactions
4. Calculations	Define the mole, convert grams to moles, **1 mole of gas = 24dm³** Percentage composition by mass of a compound, empirical vs. molecular formulae Calculate reactants in excess Calculate molar concentration: **moles = (volume cm³/1000) x concentration mol dm⁻³** Titration calculation, define saturated **Percentage yield = (actual yield/predicted yield) x 100**
5. Redox	Describe oxidation vs. reduction Recognise disproportionation Transfer of electrons, determine oxidation states
6. Bonding	Define elements vs. compounds Ionic vs. covalent vs. metallic bonding, simple and giant covalent structures
7. Groups	Alkali metals: group 1, electron donors, low melting/boiling points, store in oil, describe reaction with water, oxygen, and halogens Halogens: most reactive non-metals, establishing reactivity series with displacement reactions, reactions with silver nitrate Noble gases: least reactive elements Transition metals: position in the periodic table, properties and uses
8. Separation techniques	Compounds vs. mixtures Miscible liquid separation: fractional distillation, chromatography Immiscible liquid separation: separating funnel Dissolving, filtering, distillation, and crystallisation
9. Acids and Bases	Definitions and properties of strong and weak acids and bases
10. Rates of Reaction	Effects of concentration, temperature, particle size, catalyst presence, and pressure Calculate loss of reactant over time, predict measurable variables from chemical equation Collision theory and activation energy Function of catalysts
11. Energetics	Exothermic vs. endothermic
12. Electrolysis	Define electrode, cathode, anode, and electrolyte Why DC not AC?

	Electrolysis of brine and electroplating using copper sulfate
13. Organic	Alkanes vs. alkenes (general formulae, IUPAC terminology, saturated vs. unsaturated, combustion)
	Polymers: method of alkene polymerisation, define monomer, identify biodegradable and non-biodegradable polymers
	General formulae, chemical properties, and uses of alcohols and carboxylic acids

14. Metals	Reactivity series and displacement reactions
	Uses of common metals linked to their properties
	Extraction of metals from their ores
	Properties of transition metals including oxidation states, colour, and use as catalysts
15. Particle Theory	Describe the packing and movement of particles in all three states of matter
	Appreciate the changes in these models during a change of state (freezing, melting, evaporation, and condensation)
	Understand that the energy required is related to the bonding and structure
16. Chemical Tests	Know the benchside tests for:
	• **Hydrogen – squeaky pop**
	• **Oxygen – relight a glowing splint**
	• **Carbon dioxide – limewater turns cloudy**
	• **Chlorine – litmus paper turns red then white**
	• **Carbonates – dilute acid**
	• **Halides – silver nitrate and nitric acid**
	• **Sulfates – barium chloride and hydrochloric acid**
	Know the positive sign for metal cations in aqueous sodium hydroxide
	• Al^{3+}, Ca^{2+}, **and** Mg^{2+} **form a white precipitate**
	• Cu^{2+} **forms a blue precipitate**
	• Fe^{2+} **forms a green precipitate**
	• Fe^{3+} **forms a brown precipitate**
	Know the flame tests for cations
	• **Li – crimson red**
	• **Na – yellow-orange**
	• **K – lilac**
	• **Ca – red-orange**
	• **Cu – green**
	Test for water with anhydrous copper (II) sulfate (**white to blue**)
17. Air and Water	Fractional distillation can be used to separate the components of air
	Know the origins and effects of greenhouse gases
	Know the origins and effects of gaseous pollutants
	Know the purpose of chlorine and fluoride ions in water treatment

PHYSICS

Syllabus Point	What to Know
1. Electricity	Electrostatics: charging of insulators by friction, gain of electrons induces negative charge, uses in paint spraying and dust extraction Conductors vs. insulators **Current = charge/ time** **Resistance = voltage/ current**, how to connect ammeters and voltmeters V–I graphs for a fixed resistor and a filament lamp Series vs. parallel circuits Resistors in series (but not parallel) **Voltage = energy/ charge** Basic circuit symbols and diagrams **Power = current x voltage** **Energy = power x time**
2. Magnetism	Properties of magnets Magnetic field due to an electric current The motor effect: $\mathbf{F = BIL}$ Construction and operation of a DC motor Electromagnetic induction and the applications $\left(\dfrac{V_p}{V_s} = \dfrac{n_p}{n_s}\right)$ thus when 100% efficient $\mathbf{V_pI_p = V_sI_s}$ Method of electromagnetic induction, applied to a generator
3. Mechanics	**Speed = distance/time**, difference between speed and velocity **Acceleration = change in velocity/time** Distance-time vs. velocity-time graphs (including calculation and interpretation of gradients and average speed) Equation of motion: $\mathbf{v^2 - u^2 = 2as}$ Types of force Newtons laws: -First: **momentum = mass x velocity**, conservation of momentum -Second: **force = mass x acceleration**, **force = rate of change of momentum**, resultant force, $\mathbf{W = mg}$, gravitational field strength (~10N/kg on Earth), free fall acceleration, terminal velocity -Third = every action has an equal and opposite reaction Elastic vs inelastic extensions Hooke's law: $\mathbf{F = kx}$ Energy in a stretched sping: $\mathbf{E = \frac{1}{2}Fx = \frac{1}{2}kx^2}$ **Work = force x distance** = transfer of energy **Potential energy = mgh** **Kinetic energy** = $\frac{1}{2}\mathbf{mv^2}$ Crumple zones and road safety **Power = energy transfer/time** Conservation of energy, forms of energy, useful and wasted energy, % efficiency
4. Thermal physics	Conduction: factors affecting rate of conduction Convection: temperature and density of fluids Radiation: infrared, absorption and re-emission Experimental methods of determining densities
5. Matter	Particle models of solids, liquids, gases, and state changes Behaviour of ideal gases: **PV = constant** Understand the terms melting point, boiling point, latent heat of fusion, latent heat of vaporisation **Density = mass/volume**

Compare densities of solids, liquids, and gases

Pressure = force/area

Hydrostatic pressure = hpg

6.	**Waves**	Transfer of energy without net movement of matter, transverse (electromagnetic) vs. longitudinal (sound) Define amplitude, wavelength, frequency (1Hz = 1 wave/second), and period **Frequency = 1/period** **Wave speed = frequency x wavelength** Reflection and refraction (including ray diagrams), and Doppler effect Angle in incidence = angle of reflection Production and properties of sound waves Range of human hearing is **20Hz to 20kHz** Application of ultrasound Properties of electromagnetic waves (speed of light, transverse) Distinguished by wavelength, longest to shortest: radio, microwaves, infrared, visible light, ultraviolet, x-ray, gamma Applications and dangers
7.	**Radioactivity**	Atomic structure, charges and mass of subatomic particles, ionisation Radioactive decay: alpha vs. beta vs. gamma emission, decay equations, define activity of a sample Ionising radiation: penetrating ability, ionising ability, presence of background radiation (including origin), applications and dangers Define half-life and interpret from graphs Apply half-life calculations Nuclear fission: absorption of thermal neutrons, uranium-235 (decay equation), chain reaction Nuclear fusion: hydrogen to form helium, requires significant temperature and pressure, significance as a possible energy sauce

Section 3: An Overview

What will you be tested on?	No of Questions	Duration
The ability to select, develop and organise ideas, and to communicate them in writing, concisely and effectively.	One writing task from a choice of three questions	30 minutes

Section 3 asks you to write one A4 page essay from a choice of 3 essay questions. Obviously certain questions require some background understanding to be able to interpret the question, but essentially the only skill being tested is your ability to construct a logical and coherent argument (whether it's right or wrong does not matter).

So, the aim is not to squeeze as much as you can onto the page but rather present your opinions supported with evidence, and then tie everything together with a logical conclusion answering the initial question. Be warned that irrelevant material for the sake of filling space may actually negatively affect your score! You're scored 0 – 5 for the content of your essay and A – E for the quality of your written communication.

The theory behind the essay

Most BMAT section 3 questions all follow the same syntax. Firstly, they present a quote or statement, then ask you: 1) explain it, 2) argue for or against it, and finally 3) "to what extent" do you agree.

1) is the easy bit and shouldn't exceed three lines of text, this is your chance to lay the grounding for your essay – if you are unsure of what a word means, or the statement is ambiguous, categorically define it here and say this is what all your arguments are based around.

2) should comprise the main body of your essay. Here you need to demonstrate your understanding of the concept by offering critical insight strengthened by any evidence you are aware of. You should aim to explore two distinct ideas and acknowledge their counter arguments.

3) is really the chance for your personality to shine through. Don't be vague or unimaginative! Be brave and make a bold statement that can be derived from considering all the points you have discussed, reasoning both sides of the argument.

Structuring the essay

With such tight time constraints there is no time to devise a complex essay weaving your points through the paragraphs – and for examiners reading 100 essays a night it's just confusing. Keep it simple and follow the age old classic model described below:

Introduction: *say what you're going to say and how you're going to say it.* This is your opportunity to explain the quote/statement, give any relevant background information needed to validate your arguments, and finally indicate the logical flow of your arguments to follow.

Main body of text: *say it.* Now is the time to develop your points and insert your own personal opinions (validated by fact!) with examples if you have them. A good system to follow for each point you make is point → evidence → evaluate. Don't forget to link your paragraphs and compare arguments to show a deeper level of understanding.

Conclusion: *say what you've said.* Here you draw everything to a close. You should not introduce any new information but rather summarise your main points to leave your final take home message. Don't forget to answer the question explicitly at the end. Often a nice way to end is by asking a relevant question back to the reader that your argument brings to light.

How to use this Book

If you have done everything this book has described so far then you should be well equipped to meet the demands of the BMAT, and therefore **the mock papers in the rest of this book should ONLY be completed under exam conditions**.

This means:

➢ Absolute silence – no TV or music
➢ Absolute focus – no distractions such as eating your dinner
➢ Strict time constraints – no pausing half way through
➢ No checking the answers as you go
➢ Give yourself a maximum of three minutes between sections – keep the pressure up
➢ Complete the entire paper before marking
➢ Mark harshly

In practice this means setting aside two hours in an evening to find a quiet spot without interruptions and tackle the paper. Completing one mock paper every evening in the week running up to the exam would be an ideal target.

➢ Tackle the paper as you would in the exam.
➢ Return to mark your answers, but mark harshly if there's any ambiguity.
➢ Highlight any areas of concern.
➢ If warranted read up on the areas you felt you underperformed to reinforce your knowledge.
➢ If you inadvertently learnt anything new by muddling through a question, go and tell somebody about it to reinforce what you've discovered.

Finally relax… the BMAT is an exhausting exam, concentrating so hard continually for two hours will take its toll. So, being able to relax and switch off is essential to keep yourself sharp for exam day! Make sure you reward yourself after you finish marking your exam.

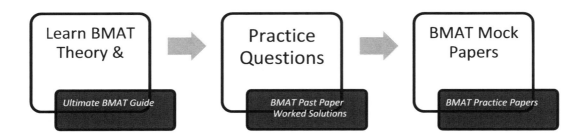

Scoring Tables

Use these to keep a record of your scores from past papers – you can then easily see which paper you should attempt next (always the one with the lowest score).

SECTION 1	1st Attempt	2nd Attempt	3rd Attempt
2003			
2004			
2005			
2006			
2007			
2008			
2009			
2010			
2011			
2012			
2013			
2014			
2015			
2016			
2017			

SECTION 2	1st Attempt	2nd Attempt	3rd Attempt
2003			
2004			
2005			
2006			
2007			
2008			
2009			
2010			
2011			
2012			
2013			
2014			
2015			
2016			
2017			

Section 3 will be much harder to mark with past papers due to the lack of example model answers to gauge yourself against. The *BMAT Past Paper Worked Solutions* book has detailed essay plans for every past paper. You can get a free copy by flicking to the back of this book.

And the same again here but with our mocks instead.

	SECTION 1	1st Attempt	2nd Attempt	3rd Attempt
Volume One	Mock A			
	Mock B			
	Mock C			
	Mock D			
Volume Two	Mock E			
	Mock F			
	Mock G			
	Mock H			

	SECTION 2	1st Attempt	2nd Attempt	3rd Attempt
Volume One	Mock A			
	Mock B			
	Mock C			
	Mock D			
Volume Two	Mock E			
	Mock F			
	Mock G			
	Mock H			

Fortunately for our mock papers our tutors have compiled model answers for you to compare your essays against! If you're repeating a mock paper, its best to attempt a different essay title to give yourself maximum experience with the various styles of BMAT essays.

	SECTION 3	Essay 1	Essay 2	Essay 3	Essay 4
Volume One	Mock A				
	Mock B				
	Mock C				
	Mock D				
Volume Two	Mock E				
	Mock F				
	Mock G				
	Mock H				

Remember! You can get a free copy of Volume 2 (Papers E to H) of *BMAT Practice Papers* by flicking to the back of this book.

MOCK PAPER A

Section 1

Question 1:

A square sheet of paper is 20cms long. How many times must it be folded in half before it covers an area of 12.5cm²?

A) 3   B) 4   (C) 5   D) 6   E) 7

Question 2:

Mountain climbing is viewed by some as an extreme sport, while for others it is simply an exhilarating pastime that offers the ultimate challenge of strength, endurance, and sacrifice. It can be highly dangerous, even fatal, especially when the climber is out of his or her depth, or simply gets overwhelmed by weather, terrain, ice, or other dangers of the mountain. Inexperience, poor planning, and inadequate equipment can all contribute to injury or death, so knowing what to do right matters.

Despite all the negatives, when done right, mountain climbing is an exciting, exhilarating, and rewarding experience. This article is an overview beginner's guide and outlines the initial basics to learn. Each step is deserving of an article in its own right, and entire tomes have been written on climbing mountains, so you're advised to spend a good deal of your beginner's learning immersed in reading widely. This basic overview will give you an idea of what is involved in a climb.

Which statement best summarises this paragraph?
A) Mountain climbing is an extreme sport fraught with dangers.
B) Without extensive experience embarking on a mountain climb is fatal.
C) A comprehensive literature search is the key to enjoying mountain climbing.
D) Mountain climbing is difficult and is a skill that matures with age if pursued.
E) The terrain is the biggest unknown when climbing a mountain and therefore presents the biggest danger.

Question 3:

50% of an isolated population contract a new strain of resistant Malaria. Only 20% are symptomatic of which 10% are female. What percentage of the total population do symptomatic males represent?

A) 1%   (B) 9%   C) 10%   D) 80%

Question 4:

John is a UK citizen yet is looking to buy a holiday home in the South of France. He is purchasing his new home through an agency. Unlike a normal estate agent, they offer monthly discount sales of up to 30%. As a French company, the agency sells in Euros. John decides to hold off on his purchase until the sale in the interest of saving money. What is the major assumption made in doing this?

A) The house he likes will not be bought in the meantime.
B) The agency will not be declared bankrupt.
C) The value of the pound will fall more than 30%.
(D) The value of the pound will fall less than 30%.
E) The value of the euro may increase by up to 35% in the coming weeks.

Question 5:

In childcare professions, by law, there must be an adult to child ratio of no more than 1:4. Child minders are hired on a salary of £8.50 an hour. What is the maximum number of children that can be continually supervised for a period of 24 hours on a budget of £1,000?

A) 1   B) 8   C) 12   D) 16   E) 468

$12 + 192$
$= 204$

Question 6:

A table of admission prices for the local cinema is shown below:

	Peak	Off-peak
Adult	£11	£9.50
Child	£7	£5.50
Concession	£7	£5.50
Student	£5	£5

How much would a group of 3 adults, 5 children, a concession and 4 students save by visiting at an off-peak time rather than a peak time?

$28.5 + 27.5$
$= 56$
61.5
81.5

$33 + 35 + 7 + 20$
$29.5 + 30 + 55 + 20$

$75 \qquad 64$

A) £11.50   B) £13.50   C) £15.50   D) £17.50   E) £18.50

Question 7:

All musicians play instruments. All oboe players are musicians. Oboes and pianos are instruments. Karen is a musician. Which statement is true?

A) Karen plays two instruments.
B) All musicians are oboe players.
C) All instruments are pianos or oboes.
D) Karen is an oboe player.
E) None of the above.

Question 8:

Flow mediated dilatation is a method used to assess vascular function within the body. It essentially adopts the use of an ultrasound scan to measure the percentage increase in the width of an artery before and after occlusion with a blood pressure cuff. Ultrasound scans are taken by one sonographer, and the average lumen diameter is then measured by an analyst. What is a potential flaw in the methodology of this technique?

A) Results will not be comparable within an individual if different arteries start at different diameters.
B) Results will not be comparable between individuals if they have different baseline arterial diameters.
C) Ultrasound is an outdated technique with no use in modern medicine.
D) This methodology is subject to human error.
E) This methodology is not repeatable.

Question 9:

If it takes 20 minutes to board an aeroplane, 15 minutes to disembark and the flight lasts two and a half hours. In the event of a delay it is not uncommon to add 20 minutes to the flight time. Megan is catching the flight in question as she needs to attend a meeting at 5pm. The location of the meeting is 15 minutes from the airport without traffic; 25 minutes with. Which of the following statements is valid considering this information?

A) If Megan wants to be on time for her meeting, given all possibilities described, the latest she can begin boarding at the departure airport is 1.30pm.
B) If Megan starts boarding at 1.40pm she will certainly be late.
C) If Megan aims to start boarding at 1.10pm she will arrive in time whether the plane is delayed or not.
D) If Megan wishes to be on time she doesn't have to worry about the plane being delayed as she can make up the time during the transport time from the arrival airport to the meeting.

Question 10:

A cask of whiskey holds a total volume of 500L. Every two and a half minutes half of the total volume is collected and discarded. How many minutes will it take for the entire cask to be emptied?

A) 80   B) 160   C) 200   D) 240   E) ∞

Question 11:

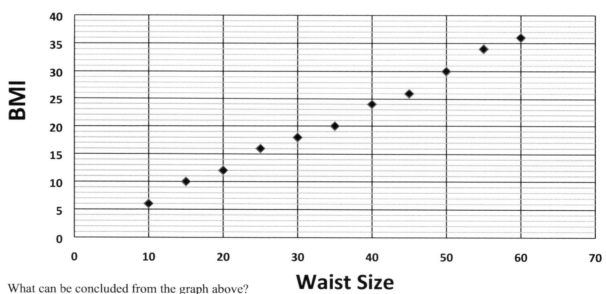

Scatter plot of Waist size vs BMI for some people

What can be concluded from the graph above?

A) Having a larger waist size causes an increase in BMI.
B) Having a larger BMI causes an increase in waist size.
C) Waist size is reciprocal to BMI.
D) No conclusions can be drawn from this graph.
E) None of the above are correct.

Question 12:

B is right of A. C is left of B. D is in front of C. E is in front of B. Where is D in relation to E?
A) D is behind E.   D) D is to the left of E.
B) E is behind D.   E) E is to the left of D.
C) D is to the right of E.

Question 13:

Car A has a fuel tank capacity of 30 gallons and achieves 40mpg. Car B on the other hand has a fuel tank capacity of 50 gallons but only achieves 30mpg. Both cars drive until they run out of fuel. If car A starts with a full tank of petrol and travels 200 miles further than car B, how full was car B's fuel tank?

A) 1/5   B) 1/4   C) 1/3   D) 1/2   E) 2/3

The information below relates to questions 14 and 15:

The art of change ringing adopts the use of 6 bells, numbered 1 to 6 in order of weight (1 being the lightest). Initially the bells are rung in this order: 1, 2, 3, 4, 5, 6 however the aim is to ultimately ring all the possible combinations of a 6-number sequence. The rules for doing this are very simple: each bell can only move a maximum of one place in the sequence every time it rings.

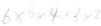

Question 14:

What is the total possible number of permutations of 6 bells?

A) 160   B) 220   C) 660   D) 720   E) 1160

Question 15:

Based on the information provided which of the following could be a possible series of bell sequences?

A) 1 2 3 4 5   B) 1 2 3 4 5   C) 1 2 3 4 5   D) 1 2 3 4 5   E) 1 2 3 4 5
    2 1 4 3 5   2 1 4 3 5   4 2 1 3 5   1 4 3 2 5   4 1 3 2 5
    2 3 1 5 4   2 4 1 5 3   4 2 3 1 5   1 2 3 4 5   5 3 1 2 4

Question 16:

The keypad to a safe comprises the digits 1 - 9. The code itself can be of indeterminate length. The code is therefore set by choosing a reference number so that when a code is entered the average of all the numbers entered must equal the chosen reference number.

Which of the following is true?

A) If the reference number was set greater than 9, the safe would be locked forever.
B) This safe is extremely insecure as if random digits were pressed for long enough it would average out at the correct reference number.
C) More than one number is always required to achieve the reference number.
D) All of the above are true.
E) None of the above are true.

Question 17:

The use of antibiotics is one of the major paradoxes in modern medicine. Antibiotics themselves provide a selection pressure to drive the evolution of antibiotic resistant strains of bacteria. This is largely due to the rapid growth rate of bacterial colonies and asexual cell division. As such a widespread initiative is in place to limit the prescription of antibiotics.
Which of the following is a fair assumption?

A) Antibiotic resistance is impossible to avoid as it is driven by evolution.
B) If bacteria reproduced at a slower rate antibiotic resistance would not be such an issue.
C) Medicine always creates more problems than it solves.
D) In the past antibiotics were used frivolously.

E)   All of the above could be possible.

The information below relates to questions 18 – 22:

The Spaghetti Bolognese recipe below serves 10 people and each portion contains 300 kcal.

➢ 1kg mince
➢ 220g pancetta, diced
➢ 30g crushed garlic

➢ 1kg tinned tomatoes
➢ 300g diced onions
➢ 300g sliced mushrooms

➢ 200g grated cheese

Question 18:
What quantity of cheese is required to prepare a meal for 350 people?

A)   0.7kg   B)   7kg   C)   70kg   D)   700kg   E)   7000kg

Question 19:
If 12 portions represent 120% of an individual's recommended calorific intake, what is that individuals recommended calorific intake?

A)   2,600kcal   B)   2,800kcal   C)   3,000kcal   D)   3,200kcal   E)   3,400kcal

Question 20:
The recommended ratio of pasta to Bolognese is 4:1. If cooking for 30 people how much pasta should be used?

A)   30.3kg   B)   36.6kg   C)   42.9kg   D)   49.2kg   E)   55.5kg

Question 21:
What is the ratio of onions to the rest of the ingredients if garlic and pancetta are ignored?

A)   1/2.05   B)   1/3.9   C)   1/6.7   D)   1/9.3   E)   1/10

Question 22:
It takes 4 minutes to prepare the ingredients per portion, and a further 8 minutes per portion to cook. Simon has ample preparation space but is limited to cooking 8 portions at a time. What is the shortest period of time it would take him to turn all the ingredients into a meal for 25 people, assuming he didn't start cooking until all the ingredients were prepared?

A)   3 hours   B)   3 hours 40   C)   4 hours   D)   4 hours 40   E)   5 hours

Question 23:
A company sells custom design t-shirts. A breakdown of their costs is shown below:

Number of Items	Cost per Item	
	Black and white	Colour
0 – 99	£3.00	£5.00
100 - 499	£2.50	£4.50
500 - 999	£2.00	£4.00
1000+	£1.00	£3.00

Customers with a never before printed design must also pay a surcharge of £50 to cover the cost of building a jig. What is the total cost for an order of unique stag do t-shirts: 50 in colour, and 200 in black and white?

A) £650   B) £700   C) £750   D) £800   E) £850

Question 24:

The Scouts is a movement for young people first established by Lord Baden Powell. As the founder he was the first chief scout of the association. Since his initial appointment there have been a number of notable chief scouts including Peter Duncan and Bear Grylls. Some of the first camping trips conducted by Lord Powell's scout troop were on Brown Sea Island.

Now the Scout movement is a worldwide global phenomenon giving children from all backgrounds the opportunity not only to embark upon adventure but also to engage in the understanding and teaching of foreign culture. Traditionally religion formed the back bone of the scouting movement which was reflected in the scouts promise: "I promise to do my duty to god and to the queen".

Which of the following applies to the scout movement?

A) Scouts work for the Queen.
B) The scout network is aimed at adventurous individuals.
C) Chief scout is appointed by the Queen.
D) You have to be religious to be a scout.
E) None of the above.

Question 25:

Three rats are placed in a maze that is in the shape of an equilateral triangle. They pick a direction at random and walk along the side of a triangle. Sophie thinks they are less likely to collide than not. Is she correct?

A) Yes, because mice naturally keep away from each other.
B) No, they are more likely to collide than not.
C) No, they are equally likely to collide than not collide.
D) Yes, because the probability they collide is 0.25.
E) None of the above.

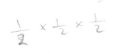

Question 26:

The use of human cadavers in the teaching of anatomy is hotly debated. Whilst many argue that it is an invaluable teaching resource, demonstrating far more than a text book can. Others describe how it is an outdated method which puts unfair stress on an already bereaved family. One of the biggest pros for using human tissue in anatomical teaching is the variation that it displays. Whilst textbooks demonstrate a standard model averaged over many 100s of specimens, many argue that it is the variation between cadavers that really reinforces anatomical knowledge.

The opposition argues that it is a cruel process that damages the grieving process of the effected family. For the use of the cadaver often occupies a period of up to 12 months. As such the relative in question is returned to the bereaved family for burial around the time it would be expected that they were recovering as described in the grieving model.

Does the article support or reject the use of cadavers in anatomical teaching?

A) Supports the use   C) Impartial   E) None of the above
B) Rejects the use   D) Can't tell

Question 27:

A ferry is carrying its full capacity. At the time of departure (7am) the travel time to the nearest hour is announced as 13 hours. What is the latest that the ferry could arrive at its destination?

A) 08.00   B) 20.00   C) 20.29   D) 20.30   E) 20.50

Question 28:

A game is played using a circle of 55 stepping stones. A die is rolled showing the numbers 1 - 6. The number on the die tells you how many steps you may take during your go. The only rule is that during your go you must take your steps in the routine two steps forward, 1 step back.

What is the minimum number or rolls required to win?

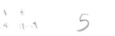

A) 28   B) 55   C) 110   D) 165   E) 200

Question 29:

On a race track there are 3 cars recording average lap times of 40 seconds, 60 seconds, and 70 seconds. They all started simultaneously 4 minutes ago. How much longer will the race need to continue for them to all cross the start line again at the same time?

A) 23.33 hours   B) 46.67 hours   C) 60.00 hours   D) 83.33 hours   E) 106.67 hours

Question 30:

A class of 60 2nd year medical students are conducting an experiment to measure the velocity of nerve conduction along their radial arteries. This work builds on a previous result obtained demonstrating the effects of how right-handed men have faster nerve conduction velocities than gender matched left handed individuals. 60% of the class are female of which 3% were unable to take part due to underlying heart conditions. 2 of the male members of the class were also unable to take part. On average the female cohort had faster nerve conduction velocities than men in their dominant arm.

Right handed women have the fastest nerve conduction velocities.

A) True   B) False   C) Can't tell

Question 31:

Mark is making a double tetrahedron dice by joining two square based pyramids together at their bases. Each square based pyramid is 5cm wide and 8cm tall. What area of card would have been required to produce the nets for the whole die?

A) 150cm^2 B) 180 cm^2 C) 210 cm^2 D) 240 cm^2 E) 270 cm^2

Question 32:

A serial dilution is performed by lining up 10 wells and filling each one with 9ml of distilled water. 1 ml of a concentrated solvent is then added to the first well and mixed. 1 ml of this new solution is drawn from the first well and added to the second and mixed. The process is repeated until all 10 wells have been used.
If the solvent starts off at concentration x, what will its final concentration be after 10 wells of serial dilution?

A) $x/10^9$ B) $x/10^{10}$ C) $x/10^{11}$ D) $x/10^{12}$ E) $x/10^{13}$

Question 33:

A student decides to measure the volume of all the blood in his body. He does this by injecting a known quantity of substrate into his arm, waiting a period of 20 minutes, then drawing a blood sample and measuring the concentration of the substrate in his blood. What assumption has he made here?

A)   The substrate is only soluble in blood.
B)   The substrate is not bioavailable.
C)   The substrate is not excreted.
D)   The substrate is not degraded.
E)   All of the above.

Question 34:

Jason is ordering a buffet for a party. The buffet company can provide a basic spread at £10 per head. However more luxurious items carry a surcharge. Jason is particularly interested in cup-cakes and shell fish. With these items included the buffet company provides a new quote of £10 per head. In addition to simply ordering the food Jason must also purchase cutlery and plates. Plates come in packs of 20 for £8 whilst cutlery is sold in bundles of 60 sets for £10.

$$10 + 0.8 + \frac{1}{6}$$

With a budget of £2,300 (to the nearest 10 people) what is the maximum number of people Jason can provide food on a plate for?

$$\frac{2300}{11} = 200$$

A) 180   B) 190   C) 209   (D) 210   E) 220

Question 35:

What were once methods of hunting have now become popular sports. Examples include archery, the javelin throw, the discus throw and even throwing a boomerang. Why such dangerous hobbies have begun to thrive is now being investigated by social scientists. One such explanation is that it is because they are dangerous we find them appealing in the first place. Others argue that it is a throwback to our ancestral heritage, where as a hunter gatherer being a proficient hunter was something to show off and flaunt. Whilst this may be the case it is well observed that many find the chase of a hunt exciting if not controversial.

Sports like archery provide excitement analogous to that of the chase during a hunter gatherer hunt.

A) True
B) False
C) Can't tell

END OF SECTION

Section 2

Question 1:

A crocodile's tail weighs 30kg. Its head weighs as much as the tail and one half of the body and legs. The body and legs together weigh as much as the tail and head combined.

What is the total weight of the crocodile?

A) 220kg   B) 240kg   C) 260kg   D) 280kg   E) 300kg

Question 2:

A body is travelling at x ms^{-1} with y J of kinetic energy. After a period of retardation the kinetic energy of the body is $1/16y$. Assuming that the mass of the body has remained constant what is its new velocity?

A) $1/196x$ B) $1/16x$ C) $1/8x$ D) $1/4x$ E) $4x$

Question 3:

Which of the following cannot be classified as an organ?

1. Blood   3. Larynx   5. Prostate   7. Skin
2. Bone   4. Pituitary Gland   6. Skeletal Muscle

A) 1 and 6   B) 2 and 3   C) 5 and 7   D) 1 and 5   E) 1,4, 5 and 6

Question 4:

An increase in aerobic respiratory rate could be associated with which of the following physiological changes?

1. A larger percentage of water vapour in expired air   4. Perspiration
2. Increased expired CO_2 5. Vasodilatation
3. Increased inspired O_2

A) 3 only   C) 1, 2 and 3 only   E) All of the above
B) 1 and 2 only   D) 2, 3 and 5

Question 5:

The nephron is to the kidney, as the _____ is to striated muscle:

A) Actin filament   D) Sarcomere
B) Artery   E) Vein
C) Myofibril

Question 6:

A diabetic patient's glucagon and insulin levels are measured over 4 hours. During this time the patient is given two large boluses of glucose. A graphical representation of this is shown right.

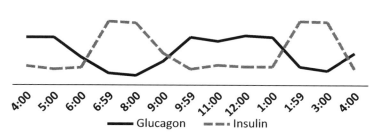

At which times would you expect the patients' blood glucose to be greatest?

A)   05:00 and 12:00   C)   08:00 and 15:00   E)   06:00, 10:00 and 16:00
B)   07:00 and 14.00   D)   10:00 and 13:00

Question 7:

In addition to the A, B or O classification, blood groups can also be distinguished by the presence of Rhesus antigen (Rh). Care must be taken in blood transfusion as once blood types are mixed a Rh -ve individual will mount an immune response against Rh +ve blood. This is particular well exemplified in haemolytic disease of the newborn – where a Rh-ve mother carries a Rh+ve foetus.

Applying what is written here and your knowledge of the human immune system, explain why the mother's first child would be relatively safe and unaffected, yet further offspring would be at high risk.

A)   The first pregnancy is always such a shock to the body it compromises the immune system. ✓
B)   Antibodies take longer than 9 months to produce and mature to an active state. ✓
C)   First born children are immunologically privileged.
D)   There is a high risk of haemorrhage to both mother and child during birth.
E)   Plasma T cells require time to multiply to lethal levels. ✓

Question 8:

Which of the following is NOT present in the Bowman's capsule?

A) Urea   C) Sodium   E) Haemoglobin
B) Glucose   D) Water

Question 9:

At present a large effort is being made to produce tailored patient care. One of the ultimate goals of this is to be able to grow personal, genetically identical organs for those with end stage organ failure. This process will first require the harbouring of what cell type?

A)   Cells from the organ that is failing   D)   Adult stem cells
B)   Haematopoietic stem cells   E)   All of the above
C)   Embryonic stem cells

Question 10:

A 1.4kg fish swims through water at a constant speed of 2ms-1. Resistive forces against the fish are 2N. Assuming g = 10ms-2, how much work does the fish do in one hour? $W = fd = 2 \times 7200$

A) 7,200 J   D) 19,880 J   F)   More information is
B) 10,080 J   E) 22,500 J   needed
C) 14,400 J

$14 \times 7200 =$

Question 11:

From which of the following elemental groups are you most likely to find a catalyst?

A)   Alkali Metals   C)   Alkaline Earth Metals   E)   Halogens
B)   d-block elements   D)   Noble Gases

$223 \overline{)1338}$

Question 12:

1.338kg of francium is mixed in a reaction vessel with an excess of distilled water. What volume will the hydrogen produced occupy at room temperature and pressure? Mr of Francium = 223

A)   20.4dm³   B) 36dm³   C) 40.8dm³   D) 60.12dm³   E) 72dm³

3×24

$\dfrac{1338}{223} =$

$2Fr + 2H_2O \rightarrow 2FrOH + H_2$

446   669   892   1115   1338

Question 13:

The composition of a compound is Carbon 30%, Hydrogen 40%, Fluorine 20%, and Chlorine 10%.
What is the empirical formula of this compound?

A) CH_2FCl

B) $C_3H_2F_2Cl$

C) C_3H_4FCl

D) $C_3H_4F_2Cl$

E) $C_4H_4F_2Cl$

Question 14:

What is the actual molecular formula of the compound in question 13 if the M_r is 340.5?

A) $C_3H_4F_2Cl$

B) $C_6H_8F_4Cl_2$

C) $C_9H_{12}F_6Cl_3$

D) $C_{12}H_{16}F_8Cl_4$

E) $C_{15}H_{20}F_{10}Cl_5$

Question 15:

1.2×10^{10} kg of sugar is dissolved in 4×10^{12} L of distilled water. What is the concentration?

A) 3×10^{-2} g/dL

B) 3×10^{-1} g/dL

C) 3×10^1 g/dL

D) 3×10^2 g/dL

E) 3×10^3 g/dL

Question 16:

Which of the following is not essential for the progression of an exothermic chemical reaction?

A)   Presence of a catalyst
B)   Increase in entropy
C)   Achieving activation energy
D)   Attaining an electron configuration more closely resembling that of a noble gas
E)   None of the above

Question 17:

What is a common use of cationic surfactants?

A)   Shampoo

B)   Lubricant

C)   Cosmetics

D)   Detergents

E)   All of the above

Question 18:

Which of the following is a unit equivalent to the Volt?

A) $A.\Omega^{-1}$

B) $J.C^{-1}$

C) $W.s^{-1}$

D) $C.s$

E) $W.C.\Omega$

Question 19:

Complete the sentence below:
A voltmeter is connected in _____ and therefore has _____ resistance; whereas an ammeter is connected in _____ and has _____ resistance.

A) Parallel, zero, parallel, infinite

B) Parallel, zero, series, infinite

C) Parallel, infinite, series, zero

D) Series, zero, parallel, infinite

E) Series, infinite, parallel, zero

Question 20:

A body "A" of mass 12kg travelling at 15m/s undergoes inelastic collision with a fixed, stationary object "B" of mass 20kg over a period of 0.5 seconds. After the collision body A has a new velocity of 3m/s. What force must have been dissipated during the collision?

A)   288N

B)   298N

C)   308N

D)   318N

E)   328N

Question 21:

What process is illustrated here: $^{14}_{6}C \rightarrow \, ^{14}_{7}N + x$

A) Thermal decomposition   C) Beta decay
B) Alpha decay   D) Gamma decay

Question 22:

A radio dish is broadcasting messages into deep space on a 20 Hz radio frequency of wavelength 3km. With every hour how much further does the signal travel into deep space? $c = 60\,000 \, m\,s^{-1}$

A) 200,000 km   C) 232,000 km   E) 264,000 km
B) 216,000 km   D) 248,000 km

$60 \times 60 \times 60$
216000

Question 23:

A formula: $\sqrt[3]{\dfrac{z(x+y)(l+m-n)}{3}}$ is given. Would you expect this formula to calculate:

A) A length   C) A volume   E) A geometric average
B) An area   D) A volume of rotation

Question 24:

Evaluate the following: $\dfrac{4.2 \times 10^{10} - 4.2 \times 10^{6}}{2 \times 10^{3}}$

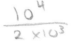

$= \dfrac{4.2 \times (10^{10} - 10^{6})}{2 \times 10^{3}}$

$1.1 \times 10^{7} - 1.1 \times 10^{3}$

A) 2.09979 x 10^6 C) 2.09979 x 10^8 E) 2.09979 x 10^{10}
B) 2.09979 x 10^7 D) 2.09979 x 10^9

$\dfrac{10^{4}}{2 \times 10^{3}}$

Question 25:

Calculate a – b

45
135

135

A) 0°
B) 5°
C) 10°
D) 15°
E) 20°

Question 26:

Jack has a bag with a complete set of snooker balls (15 red, 1 yellow, 1 green, 1 brown, 1 blue, 1 pink and 1 black ball) within it. Blindfolded Jack draws two balls from the bag.
What is the probability that he draws a blue and a black ball in any order? $\left(\dfrac{1}{21} \times \dfrac{1}{20}\right) \times 2 = \dfrac{1}{210}$

A) 2/41   B) 2/210   C) 1/210   D) 1/105   E) 2/441

Question 27:

An experiment is repeated using an identical methodology and upon further review it is proven to demonstrate identical scientific practice. If the result obtained is different to the first, this would be due to:

A) Calibration Bias   C) Random Chance
B) Systematic Bias   D) Serial dilution

E)   Inaccuracies in the methodology

END OF SECTION

Section 3

1) *Doctors should be wearing white coats as it helps produce a placebo effect making the treatment more effective.*

Explain what is meant by this statement. Argue to the contrary. To what extend do you agree with the statement? What points can you see that contradict this statement?

2) *"Medicine is a science of uncertainty and an art of probability."*

William Osler

Explain what this statement means. Argue to the contrary. To what extent do you agree with the statement?

3) *"The New England Journal of Medicine reports that 9 out of 10 doctors agree that 1 out of 10 doctors is an idiot."*

Jay Leno

What do you understand by this statement? Explain why the assumption above may be inaccurate and argue to the contrary.

4) *"My father was a research scientist in tropical medicine, so I always assumed I would be a scientist, too. I felt that medicine was too vague and inexact, so I chose physics."*

Stephen Hawking

Explain what this statement means. Argue to the contrary. To what extent do you agree with the statement?

END OF PAPER

MOCK PAPER B

Section 1

Question 1:

"If vaccinations are now compulsory because society has decided that they should be forced, then society should pay for them." Which of the following statements would weaken the argument?

A) Many people disagree that vaccinations should be compulsory.
B) The cost of vaccinations is too high to be funded locally.
C) Vaccinations are supported by many local communities and GPs.
D) Healthcare workers do not want vaccinations.
E) None of the above

Question 2:

Josh is painting the outside walls of his house. The paint he has chosen is sold only in 10L tins. Each tin costs £4.99. Assuming a litre of paint covers an area of 5m², and the total surface area of Josh's outside walls is 1050m²; what is the total cost of the paint required if Josh wants to apply 3 coats?

A)   £104.79   B)   £209.58   C)   £314.37   D)   £419.16   E)   £523.95

Question 3:

The stars of the night sky have remained unchanged for many hundreds of years, which allows sailors to navigate using the North Star still to this day. However, this only applies within the northern hemisphere as the populations of the southern hemisphere are subject to an alternative night sky.

An asterism can be used to locate the North Star, it comes by many names including the plough, the saucepan, and the big dipper. Whilst the North Star's position remains fixed in the sky (allowing it to point north reliably always) the rest of the stars traverse around the North Star in a singular motion. In a very long time, the North Star will one day move from its location due to the movement of the Earth.

Which of the following is **NOT** an assumption made in this argument?

A) The Earth is rotating on its axis.
B) Sailors still have need to navigate using the stars.
C) An analogous southern star is used to navigate in the Southern hemisphere.
D) The plough is not the only method of locating the North Star.
E) None of the above.

Question 4:

John wishes to deposit a cheque. The bank's opening times are 9am until 5pm Monday to Friday, 10am until 4pm on Saturdays, and the bank is closed on Sundays. It takes on average 42 bank hours for the money from a cheque to become available.

If John needs the money by 8pm Tuesday, what is the latest he can cash the cheque?

A) 5pm the Saturday before
B) 5pm the Friday before
C) 1pm the Thursday before
D) 1pm the Wednesday before
E) 9am the Tuesday before

Question 5:

How many different diamonds are there in the image shown to the right?

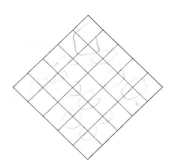

A) 25
B) 32
C) 48
D) 58
E) 63

Question 6:

In 4 years time I will be one third the age that my brother will be next year. In 20 years time he will be double my age. How old am I?

A) 4   B) 9   C) 15   D) 17   E) 23

Question 7:

Aneurysmal disease has been proven to induce systemic inflammatory effects, reaching far beyond the site of the aneurysm. The inflammatory mediator responsible for these processes remains unknown, however the effects of systemic inflammation have been well categorised and observed experimentally in pig models.

This inflammation induces an aberration of endothelial function within the inner most layer of blood vessel walls. The endothelium not only represents the lining of blood vessels but also acts as a transducer converting the haemodynamic forces of blood into a biological response. An example of this is the NO pathway, which uses the shear stress induced by increased blood flow to drive the formation of NO. NO diffuses from the endothelium into the smooth muscle surrounding blood vessels to promote vasodilatation and therefore acts to reduce blood flow.

Failure of this process induces high risk of vascular damage and therefore cardiovascular diseases such as thrombosis and atherosclerosis.

What is a valid implication from the text above?

A) Aneurysmal disease does not affect the NO pathway.
B) Aneurysms directly increase the likelihood of cardiovascular disease.
C) Aneurysms are the opposite of transducers.
D) Observations of this kind should be made in humans to see if the results can be replicated.
E) Aneurysms induce high blood flow.

Question 8:

A traffic surveyor is stood at a T-junction between a main road and a side street. He is only interested in traffic leaving the side street. He logs the class of vehicle, the colour and the direction of travel once on the main road. During an 8-hour period he observes a total of 346 vehicles including bikes. Of which 200 were travelling west whilst the rest travelled east. The over whelming majority of vehicles seen were cars at 90% with bikes, vans and articulated lorries together comprising the remaining 10%. Red was the most common colour observed whilst green was the least. Black and white vehicles were seen in equal quantities.

Which of the following is an accurate inference based on his survey?

A) Global sales are highest for those vehicles which are coloured red.
B) Cars are the most popular vehicle on all roads.
C) Green vehicle sales are down in the area that the surveyor was based.
D) The daily average rate of traffic out of a T junction in Britain is 346 vehicles over 8 hours.
E) To the east of the junction is a dead end.

Question 9:

William, Xavier, and Yolanda race in a 100m race. All of them run at a constant speed during the race. William beats Xavier by 20m. Xavier beats Yolanda by 20m. How many metres does William beat Yolanda?

A) 30m   B) 36m   C) 40m   D) 60m   E) 64m

Question 10:

A television is delivered in a box that has volume 60% larger than that of the television. The television is 150cm x 100cm x 10m. How much surplus volume is there?

A) 0.09m^2 B) 0.9 m^2 C) 9 m^2 D) 90 m^2 E) 900 m^2

Question 11:

Matthew and David are deciding where they would like to go camping Friday to Sunday. Upon completing their research, they discover the following:

➢ Whitmore Bay charges £5.50 a night and does not require a booking. The site provides showers, washing up facilities and easy access to a beach
➢ Port Eynon charges £5 a night and a booking is compulsory. However, the site does not provide showers but does have 240V sockets free of charge
➢ Jackson Bay charges £7 a night and is billed as a luxury site with compulsory booking, private showers, toilets, mobile phone charging facilities and kitchens.

David presents the following suggestion:

As Port Eynon is the farthest distance to travel the benefit of its cheap nightly rate is negated by the cost of petrol. Instead he recommends they visit Jackson Bay as it is the shortest distance to travel and will therefore be the cheapest.

Which of the following best illustrates a flaw in this argument?

A) Whitmore bay may be only a few miles further which means the total cost would be less than visiting Jackson Bay.
B) With kitchen facilities available they will be tempted to buy more food increasing the cost.
C) The campsite may be fully booked.
D) There may be a booking fee driving the cost up above that of the other campsites.
E) All of the above.

Question 12:

The manufacture of any new pharmaceutical is not permitted without scrupulous testing and analysis. This has led to the widespread, and controversial use of animal models in science. Whilst it is possible to test cyto-toxicity on simple cell cultures, to truly predict the effect of a drug within a physiological system it must be trialled in a whole organism. With animals cheap to maintain, readily available, rapidly reproducing and not subject to the same strict ethical laws they have become an invaluable component of modern scientific practice.

Which of the following best illustrates the main conclusion of this argument?

A) New pharmaceuticals cannot be approved without animal experimentation.
B) Cell culture experiments are unhelpful.
C) Modern medicine would not have achieved its current standard without animal experimentation.
D) Logistically animals are easier to keep than humans for mandatory experiments.
E) All of the above.

The information below relates to questions 13 – 17:

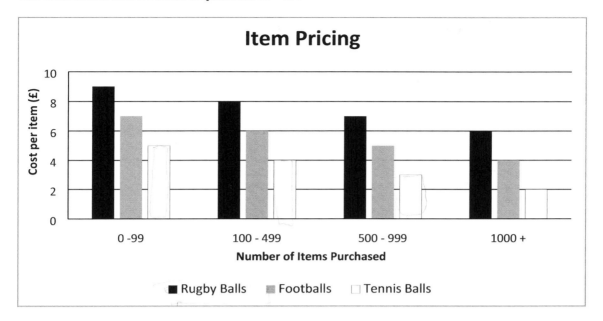

Item Pricing

The graph above shows item pricing from a wholesaler. The wholesaler is happy to deliver for a cost of £35 to companies or £5 to individuals. Any order over the cost of £100 qualifies for free delivery. Items are defined as how they come to the wholesaler therefore 1 item = 2 rugby balls or 1 football or 5 tennis balls.

Question 13:
What is the total cost to an individual purchasing 12 rugby balls and 120 tennis balls?

A) £174   B) £179   C) £208   D) £534   E) £588

6×9 + 24×5 = 120+54

Question 14:
A private gym wishes to purchase 10 of everything, how short are they of the free delivery boundary?

A) £5.00   D) £10.01
B) £5.01   E) They are already over the minimum
C) £10.00

45+ 70 +

Question 15:
What is the most number of balls that can be bought by an individual with £1,000 pounds.

A) 200   B) 250   C) 500   D) 1,000   E) 1,250

1000/4 = 333×5
250

Question 16:
The wholesaler sells all his products for a profit of 120%. If he sells £1,320 worth of goods at his prices, what did he spend on acquiring them himself?

120 1320
100 220

A) £400   B) £600   C) £800   D) £1,100   E) £1,120

220

Question 17:
If the wholesaler pays 25% tax on the amount over £12,000 pounds; how much tax does he pay when receiving an order of 2,000 of each item?   2000 × (6+4+2) = 24000

A) £2,000   B) £3,000   C) £4,000   D) £5,000   E) £6,000

Question 18:

There are four houses on a street. Lucy, Vicky, and Shannon live in adjacent houses. Shannon has a black dog named Chrissie, Lucy has a white Persian cat and Vicky has a red parrot that shouts obscenities. The owner of a four-legged pet has a blue door. Vicky has a neighbour with a red door. Either a cat or bird owner has a white door. Lucy lives opposite a green door. Vicky and Shannon are not neighbours. What colour is Lucy's door?

A) Green

B) Red

C) White

D) Blue

E) Cannot tell

Question 19:

A train driver runs a service between Cardiff and Merthyr. On average a one-way trip takes 40 minutes to drive but he requires 5 minutes to unload passengers and a further 5 minutes to pick up new ones. As the crow flies the distance between Cardiff and Merthyr is 22 miles.

Assuming he works an 8-hour shift with two 20-minute breaks, and when he arrives to work the first train is already loaded with passengers how far does he travel?

A) 132　　　　B) 143　　　　C) 154　　　　D) 176　　　　E) 198

Question 20:

The massive volume of traffic that travels down the M4 corridor regularly leads to congestion at times of commute morning and evening. A case is being made by local councils in congestion areas to introduce relief lanes thus widening the motorway in an attempt to relieve the congestion. This would involve introducing either a new 2 or 4 lanes to the motorway on average costing 1 million pound per lane per 10 miles.

Many conservationist groups are concerned as this will involve the destruction of large areas of countryside either side of the motorway. They argue that the side of a motorway is a unique habitat with many rare species residing there.

The local councils argue that with many hundreds if not thousands of cars siding idle on the motorway pumping pollutants out into the surrounding areas, it is better for the wildlife if the congestion is eased and traffic can flow through. The councils have also remarked that if congestion is eased there would be less money needed to repair the roads from car incidents with could in theory be given to the conservationist groups as a grant.

Which of the following is assumed in this passage?

A) Wildlife living on the side of the motorway cannot be re-homed.
B) Congestion causes car incidents.
C) Relief lanes have been proven to improve traffic jams.
D) A and B.
E) B and C.
F) All of the above.
G) None of the above.

Question 21:

Apples and oranges are sold in packs of 5 for the price of £1 and £1.25 respectively. Alternatively, apples can be purchased individually for 30p and oranges can be purchased individually for 50p. Helen is making a fruit salad, she remarks that her order would have cost her an extra £6.25 if she had purchased the fruit individually.

Which of the following could have been her order?

A) 15 apples 10 oranges

B) 15 apples 15 oranges

C) 25 apples 10 oranges

D) 25 apples, 15 oranges

E) 30 apples, 30 oranges

Question 22:

Janet is conducting an experiment to assess the sensitivity of a bacterial culture to a range of antibiotics. She grows the bacteria so they cover an entire Petri dish and then pipettes a single drop of differing antibiotic at different locations. A schematic of her results is shown right where black represents growth of bacteria.

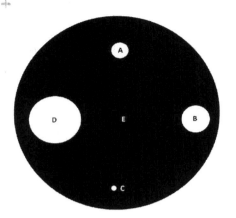

Which of the following best describes Janet's results?

A) This strain of bacteria is susceptible to all antibiotics used.

B) This strain of bacteria is susceptible to none of the antibiotics used.

C) E was the most effective antibiotic.

D) C was the most ineffective.

E) D is the most likely to be used in further testing.

Question 23:

Laura is blowing up balloons for a birthday party. The average volume of a balloon is 300cm³ and Laura's maximum forced expiratory rate in a single breathe is 4.5l/min. What is the fastest Laura could inflate 25 balloons assuming it takes her 0.5 secs to breathe in per balloon in and somebody else ties the balloons for her?

A) 112.5 seconds

B) 122.5 seconds

C) 132.5 seconds

D) 142.5 seconds

E) 152.5 seconds

Question 24:

George reasons that A is equal to B which is not equal to C. In which case C is equal to D which is equal to E. Which of the following, if true, would most *weaken* George's argument?

A) A does not equal D.

B) B is equal to E.

C) A and B are not equal.

D) C is equal to 0.

E) None of the above

Question 25:

In a single day how many times do the hour, minute and second hands of analogue clock all point to the same number?

A) 12　　　B) 24　　　C) 36　　　D) 48　　　E) 72

Question 26:

"People who practice extreme sports should have to buy private health insurance."

Which of the following statements most strongly supports this argument?

A) Exercise is healthy and private insurance offers better reward schemes.

B) Extreme spots have a higher likelihood of injury.

C) Healthcare should be free for all.

D) People that practice extreme sports are more likely to be wealthy.

Question 27:

Explorers in the US in the 18th Century had to contest with a great variety of obstacles ranging from natural to man-made. Natural obstacles included the very nature and set up of the land, presenting explorers with the sheer size of the land mass, the lack of reliable mapping as well as the lack of paths and bridges. On a human level, challenges included the threat from outlaws and other hostile groups. Due to the nature of the settling situation, availability of medical assistance was sketchy and there was a constant threat of diseases and fatal results of injuries.

Which of the following statements is correct with regards to the above text?

A) Medical supply was good in the US in the 18th Century.
B) The land was easy to navigate.
C) There were few outlaws threatening the individual.
D) Crossing rivers could be difficult.
E) All the above.

Question 28:

The statement "The human race is not dependent on electricity" assumes what?

A) We have no other energy resource.
B) Electricity is cheap.
C) Electrical appliances dominate our lives.
D) Electricity is now the accepted energy source and is therefore the only one available.
E) All of the above.

Question 29:

Wine is sold in cases of 6 bottles. A bottle of wine holds 70cl of fluid whereas a wine glass holds 175ml. Cases of wine are currently on offer for £42 a case buy one get one free. If Elin is hosting a 3-course dinner party for 27 of her friends, and she would like to provide everyone with a glass of wine per course, how much will the wine cost her?

A) £42   B) £84   C) £126   D) £168   E) £210

Question 30:

Hannah buys a television series in boxset. It contains a full 7 series with each series comprising 12 episodes. Rounded to the nearest 10 each episode lasts 40 minutes.

What is the shortest amount of time it could possibly take to watch all the episodes back to back?

A) 49 hours   B) 51 hours   C) 53 hours   D) 56 hours   E) 60 hours

Question 31:

Many are familiar with the story that aided in the discovery of the "germ". Semmelweis worked in a hospital where maternal death rates during labour were astronomically high. He noticed that medical students often went straight from dissection of cadavers to the maternity wards. As an experiment Semmelweis split the student cohort in half. Half did their maternity rotation instead before dissection whereas the other half maintained their traditional routine. In the new routine, maternity ward before dissection, Semmelweis recorded an enormous reduction in maternal deaths and thus the concept of the pathogen was born.

What is best exemplified in this passage?

A) Science is a process of trial and error.
B) Great discoveries come from pattern recognition.
C) Provision of healthcare is closely associated with technological advancements.
D) Experiments always require a control.
E) All of the above.

Question 32:

Jack sits at a table opposite a stranger. The stranger says here I have 3 precious jewels: a diamond, a sapphire, and an emerald. He tells Jack that if he makes a truthful statement Jack will get one of the stones, if he lies he will get nothing.

What must Jack say to ensure he gets the sapphire?

A)   Tell the stranger his name.
B)   Tell the stranger he must give him the sapphire.
C)   Tell the stranger he wants the emerald.
D)   Tell the stranger he does not want the emerald or the diamond.
E)   Tell the stranger he will not give him the emerald or the diamond.

Question 33:

Simon invests 100 pounds in a saver account that awards compound interest on a 6-monthly basis at 50%. Simon's current account awards compound interest on a yearly basis at 90%.

After 2 years will Simon's investment in the saver account yield more money than it would have in the current account?

A) Yes   B) No   C) Can't tell

Question 34:

My mobile phone has a 4-number pin code using the values $1 - 9$. To determine this, I use a standard algorithm of multiplying the first two numbers, subtracting the third and then dividing by the fourth. I change the code by changing the answer to this algorithm – I call this the key. What is the largest possible key?

A) 42   B) 55   C) 70   D) 80   E) 81

Question 35:

A group of scientists investigates the role of different nutrients after exercise. They set up two groups of averagely fit individuals consisting of the same number of both males and females aged $20 - 25$ and weighing between 70 and 85 kilos. Each group will conduct the same 1hr exercise routine of resistance training, consisting of various weighted movements. After the workout they will receive a shake with vanilla flavour that has identical consistency and colour in all cases. Group A will receive a shake containing 50 g of protein and 50g of carbohydrates. Group B will receive a shake containing 100 g of protein and 50 g of carbohydrates. All participants have their lean body mass measured before starting the experiment.
Which of the following statements is correct?

A)   The experiment compares the response of men and women to endurance training.
B)   The experiment is flawed as it does not take into consideration that men and women respond differently to exercise.
C)   The experiment does not consider age.
D)   The experiment mainly looks at the role of protein after exercise.
E)   None of the above.

END OF SECTION

Section 2

Question 1:

GLUT2 is an essential, ATP independent, mediator in the liver's uptake of plasma glucose. This is an example of:

A) Active transport

B) Diffusion

C) Exocytosis

D) Facilitated Diffusion

E) Osmosis

Question 2:

The molecular weight of glucose is 180 g/mol. 5.76Kg of glucose is split evenly between two cell cultures under anaerobic conditions. One cell culture is taken from human cardiac muscle, whilst the other is a yeast culture. What will be the difference (in moles) between the amount of CO_2 produced between the two cultures?

A) 0 mol   B) 4 mol   C) 8 mol   D) 12 mol   E) 16 mol

Question 3:

Which of the following cell types will have the greatest flux along endocytotic pathways?

A) Kidney cells

B) Liver cells

C) Nerve cells

D) Red blood cells

E) White blood cell

Question 4:

Compared to the Krebs cycle, the Calvin cycle demonstrates which of the following differences?

A) CO_2 as a substrate rather than a product

B) Photon dependent

C) Utilisation of different electron transporters

D) Net loss of ATP

E) All of the above

Question 5:

Pepsin and trypsin are both digestive enzymes. Pepsin acts in the stomach whereas trypsin is secreted by the pancreas. Which graph below (trypsin in black and pepsin in grey) would most accurately demonstrate their relative activity against pH?

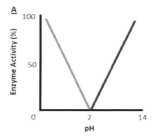
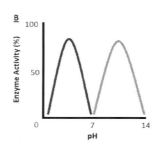
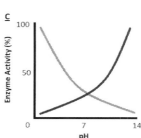

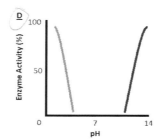
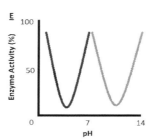

Question 6:

MRSA is an example of:

A) Natural selection
B) Genetic engineering
C) Sexual reproduction

D) Lamarckism
E) Co-dominance

Question 7:

What is the electron configuration of magnesium in $MgCl_2$?

A) 2,8
B) 2,8,2
C) 2,8,4

D) 2,8,8
E) None of the above

Mg^{2+}

Question 8:

A calcium sample is run in a mass spectrometer. It is later discovered that the sample was contaminated with the most abundant isotope of chromium. A section of the trace is shown below. What was the actual abundance of the most common calcium isotope?

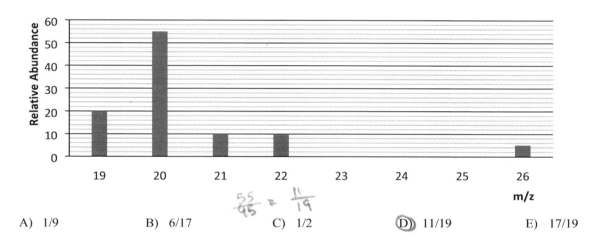

$\frac{55}{45} = \frac{11}{19}$

A) 1/9   B) 6/17   C) 1/2   D) 11/19   E) 17/19

Question 9:

A warehouse receives 15 tonnes of arsenic in bulk. Assuming that the sample is at least 80% pure, what is the minimum amount, in moles, of arsenic that they have obtained?

A) 1.6×10^5 B) 2×10^5 C) 1.6×10^6 D) 2×10^6 E) 1.6×10^7

Question 10:

A sample of silicon is run in a mass spectrometer. The resultant trace shows m/z peaks at 26 and 30 with relative abundance 60% and 30% respectively. What other isotope of silicon must have been in the sample to give an average atomic mass of 28?

$\frac{156 + 90 + x}{10} = 28$ 190

A) 28   B) 30   C) 32   D) 34   E) 36

Question 11:

72.9g of pure magnesium ribbon is mixed in a reaction vessel with the equivalent of 54g of steam. The ensuing reaction produces $72dm^3$ of hydrogen. Which of the following statements is true?

A) This is a complete reaction
B) This is a partial reaction
C) There is an excess of steam

D) There is an excess of magnesium
E) Magnesium hydroxide is a product

Question 12:

Which species is the reducing agent in: $3Cu^{2+} + 3S^{2-} + 8H^+ + 8NO_3^- \rightarrow 3Cu^{2+} + 3SO_4^{2-} + 8NO + 4H_2O$

A) Cu^{2+} B) S^{2-} C) H^+ D) NO_3^- E) H_2O

Question 13:

Which of the following is not true of alkanes?

A) C_nH2_{n+2}
B) Saturated
C) Reactive
D) Produce only CO_2 and water when burnt in an excess of oxygen
E) None of the above

Question 14:

A rubber balloon is inflated and rubbed against a sample of animal fur for a period of 15 seconds. At the end of this process the balloon is carrying a charge of -5 coulombs. What magnitude of current must have been induced during the process of rubbing the balloon against the animal fur; and in which direction was it flowing?

A) 0.33A into the balloon
B) 0.33A into the fur
C) 0.33A in no net direction
D) 75A into the balloon
E) 75A into the fur

Question 15:

Which of the following is a unit equivalent to the Amp?

A) $V.\Omega$ B) $(W.V)/s$ C) $C.\Omega$ D) $(J.s^{-1})/V$ E) $C.s$

Question 16:

The output of a step-down transformer is measured at 24V and 10A. Given that the transformer is 80% efficient what must the initial power input have been?

A) 240W   B) 260W   C) 280W   D) 300W   E) 320W

Question 17:

An electric winch system hoists a mass of 20kg 30 metres into the air over a period of 20 seconds. What is the power output of the winch assuming the system is 100% efficient?

A) 100W   B) 200W   C) 300W   D) 400W   E) 500W

Question 18:

6×10^{10} atoms of a radioactive substance remain. The activity of the substance is quantified as 3.6×10^9. What is the decay constant of this material?

A) 0.00006   B) 0.0006   C) 0.006   D) 0.06   E) 0.6

Question 19:

An 80W filament bulb draws 0.5A of household electricity. What is the efficiency of the bulb?

A) 25%   B) 33%   C) 50%   D) 66%   E) 75%

Question 20 :

$$x = \frac{\sqrt{b^3 - 9st}}{13j} + \int_{-z}^{z} 9a - 7$$

Rearrange the following equation in terms of t:

A) $t = \dfrac{(13jx - \int_{-z}^{z} 9a - 7)^2 - b^3}{9s}$

B) $t = \dfrac{13jx^2}{b^3 - 9s} - \int_{-z}^{z} 9a - 7$

C) $t = x - \dfrac{\sqrt{b^3 - 9s}}{13j} - \int_{-z}^{z} 9a - 7$

D) $t = \dfrac{x^2}{\dfrac{b^3 - 9s}{13j} + \int_{-z}^{z} 9a - 7}$

E) $t = \dfrac{[13j(x - \int_{-z}^{z} 9a - 7)]^2 - b^3}{-9s}$

(handwritten working:)
$4.5e^2 - 7z - 4.5z^2 = 7z$
$x = \dfrac{\sqrt{b^3 - 9st}}{130} - 14z$
$13\sqrt{x} = \sqrt{b^3 - 9st} - 1822\sqrt{}$
$(13\sqrt{x} + 1822\sqrt{})^2$
$b^3 - \dfrac{(13j(x - \int 9a - 7))^2}{9s}$

Question 21:

In a healthy person, which one of the following has the highest blood pressure?

A) The vena cava
B) The systemic capillaries
C) The pulmonary artery
D) The pulmonary vein
E) The aorta
F) The coronary artery

Question 22:

What is the equation of the line of best fit for the scatter graph below?

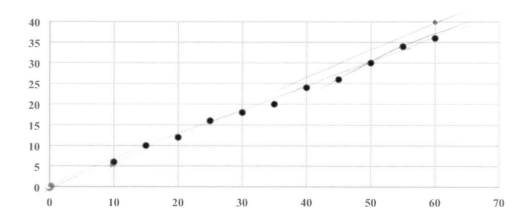

A) y = 0.2x + 0.35
B) y = 0.2x − 0.35
C) y = 0.4x + 0.35
D) y = 0.4x − 0.35
E) y = 0.6x + 0.35

Question 23 :

$$m = \sqrt{\frac{9xy^3z^5}{3x^9yz^4} - m}$$

Simplify:

A) $m = \sqrt{\frac{3y^2z}{x^8} - m}$

B) $m^2 = \frac{3y^2z}{x^8} - m$

C) $2m = \sqrt{\frac{3y^2z}{x^8}}$

D) $2m^2 = 3x^{-8}y^2z$

E) $4m^2 = 3x^{-8}y^2z$

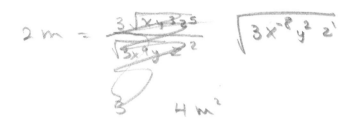

Question 24:
Which of the following is a suitable descriptive statistic for non-normally distributed data?

A) Mean
B) Normal range
C) Confidence interval

D) Interquartile range
E) Mode

Question 25:
Which best describes the purpose of statistics?

A) Evaluate acceptable scientific practice.
B) Reduce the ability of others to criticise the data
C) To quickly analyse data
D) Calculate values representative of the population from a subset sample
E) To allow for universal comparison of scientific methods

Question 26:
A rotating disc has two wells, in which bacteria are cultured. The first well is 10 cm from the centre whereas the second well is 20 cm from the centre. If the inner well completes a revolution in 1 second, how much faster is the outer well travelling?

A) 0.314m/s   B) 0.628m/s   C) 0.942m/s   D) 1.256m/s   E) 1.590m/s

Question 27:

Which is the equivalent function to: $y = 9x^{-\frac{1}{3}}$?

A) $y = \dfrac{1}{x}$

B) $y = \sqrt[3]{9x}$

C) $y = \dfrac{1}{\sqrt[3]{9x}}$

D) $y = \dfrac{9}{\sqrt[3]{x}}$

E) $y = \dfrac{3}{\sqrt[3]{x}}$

END OF SECTION

Section 3

1) *"Progress is made by trial and failure; the failures are generally a hundred times more numerous than the successes; yet they are usually left unchronicled."*

Williams Ramsey

Explain what this statement means. Argue to the contrary. To what extent do you agree with the statement?

2) *"He who studies medicine without books sails an uncharted sea, but he who studies medicine without patients does not go to sea at all."*

William Osler

Explain what this statement means. Argue to the contrary. To what extent do you agree with the statement?

3) *'"Medicine is the restoration of discordant elements; sickness is the discord of the elements infused into the living body"*

Leonardo da Vinci

Explain what this statement means. Argue to the contrary. To what extent do you think this simplification holds true within modern medicine?

4) *"Modern medicine is a negation of health. It isn't organized to serve human health, but only itself, as an institution. It makes more people sick than it heals."*

Ivan Illich

What does this statement mean? Argue to the contrary, that the primary duty of a doctor is not to prolong life. To what extent do you agree with this statement?

END OF PAPER

MOCK PAPER C

Section 1

Question 1:

Adam, Beth and Charlie are going on holiday together. A single room costs £60 per night, a double room costs £105 per night and a four-person room costs £215 per night. It is possible to opt out from the cleaning service and to pay £12 less each night per room.

What is the minimum amount the three friends could pay for their holiday for a three-night stay at the hotel?

A) £122   B) £144   C) £203   D) £423   E) £432

Question 2:

I have two 96ml glasses of squash. The first is comprised of $\frac{1}{6}$ squash and $\frac{5}{6}$ water. The second is comprised of $\frac{1}{4}$ water and $\frac{3}{4}$ squash. I take 48ml from the first glass and add it to glass two. I then take 72ml from glass two and add it to glass one.

How much squash is now in each glass?

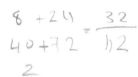
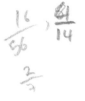

A) 16ml squash in glass one and 72ml squash in glass two.
B) 40ml squash in glass one and 32ml squash in glass two.
C) 48ml squash in glass one and 32ml squash in glass two.
D) 48ml squash in glass one and 40ml squash in glass two.
E) 80ml squash in glass one and 40ml squash in glass two.

Question 3:

It may amount to millions of pounds each year of taxpayers' money; however, it is strongly advisable for the HPV vaccination in schools to remain. The vaccine, given to teenage girls, has the potential to significantly reduce cervical cancer deaths and furthermore, the vaccines will decrease the requirement for biopsies and invasive procedures related to the follow-up tests. Extensive clinical trials and continued monitoring suggest that both Gardasil and Cervarix are safe and tolerated well by recipients. Moreover, studies demonstrate that a large majority of teenage girls and their parents are in support of the vaccine.

Which of the following is the conclusion of the above argument?

A) HPV vaccines are safe and well tolerated
B) It is strongly advisable for the HPV vaccination in schools to remain
C) The HPV vaccine amounts to millions of pounds each year of taxpayers' money
D) The vaccine has the potential to significantly reduce cervical cancer deaths
E) Vaccinations are vital to disease prevention across the population

Question 4:

Anna cycles to school, which takes 30 minutes. James takes the bus, which leaves from the same place as Anna, but 6 minutes later and gets to school at the same time as Anna. It takes the bus 12 minutes to get to the post office, which is 3km away. The speed of the bus is $\frac{5}{4}$ the speed of the bike. One day Anna leaves 4 minutes late.

How far does she get before she is overtaken by the bus?

A) 1.5km   B) 2km   C) 3km   D) 4km   E) 6km

Question 5:

The set two maths teacher is trying to work out who needs to be moved up to set one and who to award a certificate at the end of term. The students must fulfil certain criteria:

Reward	Criteria
Move to set one	Attendance over 95%
	Average test mark over 92
	Less than 5% homework handed in late
Awarded a Certificate	Absences below 4%
	Average test mark over 89
	At least 98% homework handed in on time

	Terry	Alex	Bahara	Lucy	Shiv
Attendance %	97	92	97	100	98
Average test mark %	89	93	94	95	86
Homework handed in on time %	96	92	100	96	98

Who would move up a set and who would receive a certificate?

A) Bahara would move up a set and receive a certificate.
B) Bahara and Lucy would move up a set and Bahara would receive a certificate.
C) Bahara, Terry and Lucy would move up a set and Bahara and Shiv would receive a certificate.
D) Lucy would move up a set and Bahara would receive a certificate.
E) Lucy would move up a set and Bahara and Terry would receive a certificate.

Question 6:

18 years ago, A was 25 years younger than B is now. In 21 years time, A will be 28 years older than B was 14 years ago. How old is A now if A is $\frac{5}{6}$B?

A) 27   B) 28   C) 35   D) 42   E) 46

Question 7:

The time now is 10.45am. I am preparing a meal for 16 guests who will arrive tomorrow for afternoon tea. I want to make 3 scones for each guest, which can be baked in batches of 6. Each batch takes 35 minutes to prepare and 25 minutes to cook in the oven and I can start the next batch while the previous batch is in the oven. I also want to make 2 cupcakes for each guest, which can be baked in batches of 8. It takes 15 minutes to prepare the mixture for each batch and 20 minutes to cook them in the oven. I will also make 3 cucumber sandwiches for each guest. 6 cucumber sandwiches take 5 minutes to prepare.

What will the time be when I finish making all the food for tomorrow?

A) 4:35pm   B) 5.55pm   C) 6:00pm   D) 6:05pm   E) 7:20pm

Question 8:

Pyramid	Base edge (m)	Volume (m ^{3})
1	3	33
2	4	64
3	2	8
4	6	120
5	2	8
6	6	120
7	4	64

What is the difference between the height of the smallest and tallest pyramids?

A) 1m   B) 5m   C) 4m   D) 6m   E) 8m

Question 9:

The wage of Employees at Star Bakery is calculated as: £210 + (Age x 1.2) – 0.8 (100 - % attendance).
Jessica is 35 and her attendance is 96%. Samira is 65 and her attendance is 89%.

What is the difference between their wages?

A) £30.40   B) £60.50   C) £248.80   D) £263.20   E) £279.20

Question 10:

It is important that research universities demonstrate convincing support of teaching. Undergraduates comprise an overwhelming proportion of all students and universities should make an effort to cater to the requirements of the majority of their student body. After all, many of these students may choose to pursue a path involving research and a strong education would provide students with skills equipped towards a career in research.

What is the conclusion of the above argument?

A) Undergraduates comprise an overwhelming proportion of all students.
B) A strong education would provide a strong foundation and skills equipped towards a career in research.
C) Research universities should strongly support teaching.
D) Institutions should provide undergraduates with a high-quality learning experience.
E) Research has a greater impact than teaching and limited universities funds should mainly be invested in research.

Question 11:

American football has reached a level of violence that puts its players at too high a level of risk. It has been suggested that the NFL, the governing body for American football should get rid of the iconic helmets. The hard-plastic helmets all have to meet minimum impact-resistance standards intended to enhance safety, however in reality they gave players a false sense of security that only resulted in harder collisions. Some players now suffer from early onset dementia, mood swings and depression. The proposal to ban helmets for good should be supported. Moreover, it would prevent costly legal settlements involving the NFL and ex-players suffering from head trauma.

What is the conclusion of the above argument?

A) Sports players should not be exposed to unnecessary danger.
B) Helmets give players a false sense of security.
C) Players can suffer from early onset dementia, mood swings and depression.
D) The proposal to ban helmets should be supported.
E) American football is too violent and puts its players at risk.

Question 12:

At the final stop (stop 6), 10 people get off the tube. At the previous stop (stop 5) $\frac{1}{2}$ of passengers got off. At stop 4, $\frac{3}{5}$ of passengers got off. At stop 3, $\frac{1}{3}$ of passengers got off and at stops 1 and 2, $\frac{1}{6}$ of passengers got off.

How many passengers got on at the first stop?

A) 10   B) 36   C) 90   D) 108   E) 3600

Question 13:

Everyone likes English. Some students born in spring like Maths and some like Biology. All students born in winter like Music and some like Art. Of those born in autumn, no one likes Biology, and everyone likes Art.

Which of the following is true?

A) Some students born in spring like both Biology and Maths.
B) Students born in spring, winter, and autumn all like Art.
C) No one born in winter or autumn likes Biology.
D) No one who likes Biology also likes Art.
E) Some students born in winter like 3 subjects.

Question 14:

Until the twentieth century, the whole purpose of art was to create beautiful, flawless works. Artists attained a level of skill and craft that took decades to perfect and could not be mirrored by those who had not taken great pains to master it. The serenity and beauty produced from movements such as impressionism has however culminated in repulsive and horrific displays of rotting carcasses designed to provoke an emotional response rather than admiration. These works cannot be described as beautiful by either the public or art critics. While these works may be engaging on an intellectual or academic level, they no longer constitute art.

Which of the following is an assumption of the above argument?

A) Beauty is a defining property of art.
B) All modern art is ugly.
C) Twenty first century artists do not study for decades.
D) The impressionist movement created beautiful works of art.
E) Some modern art provokes an emotional response.

Question 15:

The cost of sunglasses is reduced over the bank holiday weekend. On Saturday, the price of the sunglasses on Friday is reduced by 10%. On Sunday the price of the sunglasses on Saturday is reduced by 10%. On Monday, the price of the sunglasses on Sunday is reduced by a further 10%. What percentage of the price on Friday is the price of the sunglasses on Monday?

A) 55.12%   B) 59.10%   C) 63.80%   D) 70.34%   E) 72.9%

Question 16:

Putting the digit 7 on the right-hand side of a two-digit number causes the number to increase by 565. What is the value of the two-digit number?

A) 27   B) 52   C) 62   D) 66   E) 627

Question 17:

When folded, which box can be made from the net shown below?

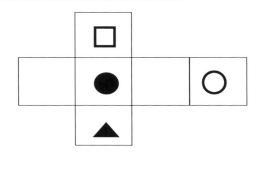

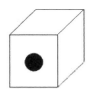 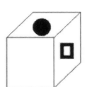 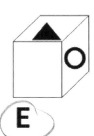

A   **B**   **C**   **D**   **E**

Question 18:

The grid is comprised of 49 squares. The shape's area is 588cm². What is its perimeter in cm?

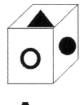

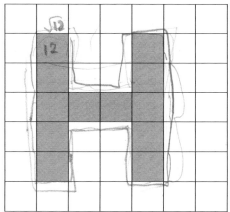

A) 26   B) 49   C) 84   D) 126   E) 182

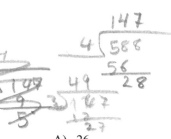
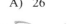

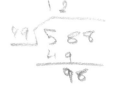

Questions 19-21 refer to the following information:

$$BMI = weight\ (kg)\ \div\ height^2\ (m^2)$$

Men	BMR= (10 x weight in kg) + (6.25 x height in cm) – (5 x age in years) + 5
Women	BMR= (10 x weight in kg) + (6.25 x height in cm) – (5 x age in years) -161

Recommended Intake:

Amount of Exercise	Daily Kilocalories required
Little to no exercise	BMR x 1.2
Light exercise 1-3 days per week	BMR x 1.375
Moderate exercise 3-5 days per week	BMR x 1.55
Heavy exercise 6-7 days per week	BMR x 1.725
Very heavy exercise twice per day	BMR x 1.9

Question 19:
A child weighs 35kg and is 120cm tall. What is the BMI of the child to the nearest two decimal places?

A) 0.0024   B) 24.28   C) 24.31   D) 42.01   E) 42.33

Question 20:
What is the BMR of a 32-year-old woman weighing 80kg and measuring 1.7m in height?

A) 643.7 kcal   B) 1537 kcal   C) 1541.5 kcal   D) 1707.5 kcal   E) 2707.5 kcal

Question 21:
What is the recommended intake of a 45-year-old man weighing 80kg and measuring 1.7m in height who does little to no exercise each week?

A) 1642.5 kcal   B) 1771.8 kcal   C) 1851 kcal   D) 1971 kcal   E) 2712.5 kcal

Questions 22 and 23 relate to the following passage:
The achievement levels of teenagers could be higher if school started later. Teenagers are getting too little sleep because they attend schools that start at 8:30am or earlier. A low level of sleep disrupts the body's circadian rhythms and can contribute to health problems such as obesity and depression. Some doctors are now urging schools to start later in order for teenagers to get sufficient sleep; ideally 8.5 to 9.5 hours each night. During adolescence, the hormone melatonin is released comparatively later in the day and the secretion levels climb at night. Consequently, teenagers can have trouble getting to sleep earlier in the night before sufficient melatonin is present. A school in America tested this idea by starting one hour later and the percentage of GCSEs at grades A* - C increased by 16%. Schools in the UK should follow by example and shift start times later.

Question 22:
Which of the following is a flaw in the above argument?

A) Slippery slope.
B) Hasty generalisation.
C) It confuses correlation with cause.
D) Circular argument.
E) Schools should not prioritise academic achievement.

Question 23:

Which of the following, if true, would most strengthen the above argument?

A) Teenagers who are more alert will disrupt the class more.
B) Getting more sleep at night is proven to increase activity levels.
C) American schools and British schools teach the same curriculum.
D) The school in America did not alter any other aspects of the school during the trial for example curriculum, teachers, and number of students in each class.
E) Teachers get tired towards the end of the school day and are less effective.

Question 24:

The UK energy market is highly competitive. In an effort to attract more business and increase revenue, the company EnergyFirst has invested significant funds into its publicity sector. Last month, they doubled their advertising expenditures, becoming the energy company to invest the greatest proportion of investment into advertising. As a result, it is expected that EnergyFirst will expand its customer base at a rate exceeding its competitors in the ensuing months. Other energy companies are likely to follow by example.

Which of the following, if true, is most likely to weaken the above argument?

A) Other companies invest more money into good customer service.
B) Research into the energy industry demonstrates a low correlation between advertising investment and new customers.
C) The UK energy market is not highly competitive.
D) EnergyFirst currently has the smallest customer base.
E) Visual advertising heavily influences customers.

Question 25:

The consumption of large quantities of red meat is suggested to have negative health ramifications. Carnitine is a compound present in red meat and a link has been discovered between carnitine and the development of atherosclerosis, involving the hardening, and narrowing of arteries. Intestinal bacteria convert carnitine to trimethylamine-N-oxide, which has properties that are damaging to the heart. Moreover, red meat consumption has been associated with a reduced life expectancy. It may be that charring meat generates toxins that elevate the chance of developing stomach cancer. If people want to be healthy, a vegetarian diet is preferable to a diet including meat. Vegetarians often have lower cholesterol and blood pressure and a reduced risk of heart disease.

Which of the following is an assumption of the above argument?

A) Diet is essential to health and we should all want to be healthy.
B) Vegetarians do the same amount of exercise as meat eaters.
C) Meat has no health benefits.
D) People who eat red meat die earlier.
E) Red meat is the best source of iron.

Question 26:

Auckland is 11 hours ahead of London. Calgary is 7 hours behind London. Boston is 5 hours behind London. The flight from Auckland to London is 22 hours, but the plane must stop for 2 hours in Hong Kong. The flight from London to Calgary is 8 hours 30 minutes. The flight from Calgary to Boston is 6 hours 30 minutes. Sam leaves Auckland at 10am for London. On arrival to London, he waits 3 hours then gets the plane to Calgary. Once in Calgary, he waits 1.5 hours and gets the plane to Boston. What time is it when Sam arrives in Boston?

A) 13:30pm   B) 22.30pm   C) 01:00am   D) 01:30am   E) 03:30am

Question 27:

Light A flashes every 18 seconds, light B flashes every 33 seconds and light C flashes every 27 seconds. The three lights all flashed at the same time 5 minutes ago.

How long will it be until they next all flash simultaneously?

A) 33 seconds   B) 294 seconds   C) 300 seconds   D) 333 seconds   E) 594 seconds

Question 28:

There are 30 students in a class. They must all play at least 1 instrument, but no more than 3 instruments. 70% play the piano, 40% play the violin, 20% play the guitar and 10% play the saxophone. Which of the following statements must be true?

1. 3 or more students play piano and violin.
2. 12 students or less play the piano and the violin.
3. 9 or more students do not play piano or violin.

A) 1 only   B) 1 and 2   C) 2 only   D) 2 and 3   E) 3 only

Question 29:

Neil, Simon and Lucy are playing a game to see who can role the highest number with two dice. They start with £50 each. The losers must halve their money and give it to the winner of each game. If it is a draw, the two winners share the loser's money. If all three tie, then they keep their money. Neil wins game 1, Simon and Lucy win game 2 and 5 and Lucy wins games 3 and 4.

How much money does Lucy gain?

A) £15.63   B) £75.00   C) £75.16   D) £78.13   E) £128.10

Question 30:

Drivers in the age group 17-19 comprise 1.5% of all drivers; however, 12% of all collisions involve young drivers in this age category. The RAC Foundation wants a graduated licensing system with a 1-year probationary period with restrictions on what new drivers can do on roads. Additionally, driving instructors need to emphasise the dangers of driving too fast and driving tests should be designed to make new drivers more focused on noticing potential hazards. These changes are essential and could stop 4,500 injuries on an annual basis.

What is the assumption of the above argument?

A) Young drivers are more likely to have more passengers than other age groups.
B) Young drivers spend more hours driving than older drivers.
C) Young drivers are responsible for the collisions.
D) The cars that young people drive are unsafe.
E) Most young drivers involved in accidents are male.

Question 31:

The mean weight of 6 apples is 180g. The lightest apple weighs 167g. What is the highest possible weight of the heaviest apple?

A) 193g   B) 225g   C) 235g   D) 245g   E) 255g

Question 32:

"Sugar should be taxed like alcohol and cigarettes."

Which of the following arguments most supports this claim?

A) Sugar can cause diabetes.
B) Sugar has high addictive potential and is associated with various health concerns.
C) High sugar diets increase obesity.
D) People that eat a lot of sugar are more likely to start abusing alcohol.
E) None of the above.

Question 33:

The farmer had 184 sheep to sell. He intended to sell each for £112. However, he sold less than one quarter on day 1. As a result, he reduced the price by $\frac{1}{8}$. On the second day he sold twice as many and made £3528 more than on day 1, leaving him with less than $\frac{1}{3}$ of original. How many sheep did he sell altogether?

A) 42   B) 84   C) 98   D) 112   E) 1

Question 34:

There is no empirical evidence that human activities directly result in global warming and this is used as a reason against decreasing carbon emissions. However, many scientists believe that human activity is highly likely to cause global warming since higher levels of greenhouse gases cause the atmosphere to thicken, retaining heat. It therefore seems sensible that we should not wait for proof considering the catastrophic effects of climate change, regardless of subsequent findings. Similarly, if a tree branch had a significant chance of falling on you, it would be sensible to move away immediately.

What is the main conclusion?

A) Many scientists believe that human activity is highly likely to cause global warming.
B) We should not wait for proof of climate change.
C) If a tree branch had a significant chance of falling on you, it would be sensible to move away immediately.
D) The effects of climate change are catastrophic.
E) There is no empirical evidence that human activities directly result in global warming, so we should not reduce carbon emissions.

Question 35:

The average of 8 numbers is y. If 13 and 31 are added, the mean of the 10 numbers is also y. What is y?

A) 11   B) 22   C) 25   D) 27   E) 44

END OF SECTION

Section 2

Question 1:
Which of the following are correct regarding polymers?

1. Sucrose is formed by the condensation of hundreds of monosaccharides.
2. Lactose is found in milk and is formed by condensation of two glucose molecules.
3. Glucose has two isomers.
4. Glycogen, starch and cellulose are all polysaccharides formed by condensation of multiple glucose molecules.
5. People with lactose intolerance lack lactase and can experience diarrhoea after drinking milk.

A) 1 only   D) 3, 4 and 5
B) 1, 2 and 3   E) 4 and 5 only
C) 1 and 3 only

Question 2:
Which of the following statements regarding enzymes are correct?

1. Enzymes are denatured at high temperatures or extreme pH values.
2. Amylase is produced in the salivary glands only and converts starch to sugars.
3. Lipases catalyse the breakdown of oils and fats into glycerol and fatty acids. This takes place in the small intestine.
4. Bile is stored in the pancreas and travels down the bile duct to neutralise stomach acid.
5. Isomerase can be used to convert glucose into fructose for use in slimming products.

A) 1 and 3 only   D) 2 and 4 only
B) 1, 3 and 4 only   E) 3 and 5 only
C) 1, 3 and 5

Question 3:
Which of the following describes the role of the colon?

A) Food is combined with bile and digestive enzymes.
B) Storage of faeces.
C) Reabsorption of water.
D) Faeces leave the alimentary canal.
E) Any digested food is absorbed into the lymph and blood.

Question 4:
Which of the following are true?

1. A nerve impulse is transmitted along the nerve axon as an electrical impulse and across the synapse by diffusion of chemical neurotransmitters.
2. Drugs that block synaptic transmission can cause complete paralysis.
3. The fatty sheath around the axon slows the speed at which nerve impulses are transmitted.
4. The peripheral nervous system includes the brain and spinal cord.
5. A reflex arc bypasses the brain and enables a fast, autonomic response.

A) 1 and 2   D) 2, 4 and 5
B) 1, 2 and 3   E) 3, 4 and 5
C) 1, 2 and 5

Question 5:
Which of the following statements are true regarding the transition elements?
1. Iron (II) compounds are light green.
2. Transition elements are neither malleable nor ductile.
3. Transition metal carbonates may undergo thermal decomposition.
4. Transition metal hydroxides are soluble in water.
5. When Cu^{2+} ions are mixed with sodium hydroxide solution, a blue precipitate is formed.

A) 1 and 2   B) 1 and 3   C) 1, 3 and 5   D) 3 and 5   E) 5 only

Question 6:
What is the value of C when the equation is balanced?

$$5\,PhCH_3 + 4\,KMnO_4 + 9\,H_2SO_4 = 5\,PhCOOH + B\,K_2SO_4 + C\,MnSO_4 + 14\,H_2O$$

A) 3   B) 4   C) 5   D) 7   E) 9

Question 7:
Tongue-rolling is controlled by the dominant allele T, while non-rolling is controlled by the recessive allele, t. Red-green colour blindness is controlled by a sex-linked gene on the X chromosome. Normal colour vision is controlled by dominant allele B, while red-green colour blindness is controlled by the recessive allele, b.
The mother of a family is colour blind and heterozygous for tongue-rolling, while the father has normal colour vision and is a non-roller.

Which of the following statements are correct?

1. More males than females in a population are red-green colour blind.
2. 50% of children will be non-rollers.
3. All the male children will be colour-blind.

A) 1 and 2 only   D) 2 and 3 only
B) 1, 2 and 3   E) 3 only
C) 2 only

Question 8:

Make y the subject of the formula: $\dfrac{y+x}{x} = \dfrac{x}{a} + \dfrac{a}{x}$

A) $y = \dfrac{x^2}{a} + a$

B) $y = \dfrac{x^2 + a^2 - ax}{a}$

C) $y = \dfrac{-ax}{x^2 + a^2}$

D) $y = \dfrac{x^2}{ax} + a - x$

E) $y = a^2 - ax$

Question 9:
What is the mass in grams of calcium chloride, $CaCl_2$, in $25cm^3$ of a solution with a concentration of $0.1\ mol.l^{-1}$? (Ar of Ca is 40 and Ar of Cl is 35)

A) 0.28g   B) 0.46g   C) 0.48g   D) 0.72g   E) 1.28g

Question 10:
A ball of mass 5kg is at rest at the top of a 5m slope. Calculate the velocity of the ball as it travels down the slope. Take $g = 10kgm^{-1}$ and assume there is no resistance.

A) 10   B) 45   C) 100   D) 5   E) 6

Question 11:
Which of the following statements regarding the circulatory system are correct?

1. The pulmonary artery carries oxygenated blood from the right ventricle to the lungs.
2. The aorta has a high content of elastic tissue and carries oxygenated blood from the left ventricle around the body.
3. The mitral valve is between the pulmonary vein and the left atrium.
4. The vena cava carries deoxygenated blood from the body to the right atrium.

A) 1 and 3   B) 1 and 2   C) 2 only   D) 2 and 4   E) 3 only

Question 12:
A compound with a molar mass of 120 g.mol^{-1} contains 12g of carbon, 2g of hydrogen and 16g oxygen. What is the molecular formula of the compound?

A) CH_2O B) $C_2H_4O_2$ C) C_4H_2O D) $C_4H_8O_4$ E) $C_8H_{16}O_8$

Question 13:
Which of the following statements, regarding normal human digestion, is FALSE?

A) Amylase is an enzyme which breaks down starch
B) Amylase is produced by the pancreas
C) Bile is stored in the gallbladder
D) The small intestine is the longest part of the gut
E) Insulin is released in response to feeding
F) None of the above

Question 14:
What is the median of the following numbers: $\frac{7}{36}$; $0.\overset{.}{3}$; $\frac{11}{18}$; 0.25; 0.75; $\frac{62}{72}$; $\frac{7}{7}$

A) $\frac{7}{36}$
B) $0.\overset{.}{3}$
C) $\frac{11}{18}$
D) $\frac{62}{72}$
E) 0.75

Question 15:
16.4g of nitrobenzene is produced from 13g of benzene in excess nitric acid: $C_6H_6 + HNO_3 \rightarrow C_6H_5NO_2 + H_2O$

What is the percentage yield of nitrobenzene ($C_6H_5NO_2$)?

A) 65%   B) 67%   C) 72%   D) 78%   E) 80%

Question 16:
Which of the following points regarding electromagnetic waves are correct?

1. Radiowaves have the longest wavelength and the lowest frequency.
2. Infrared has a shorter wavelength than visible light and is used in optical fibre communication, and heater and night vision equipment.
3. All of the waves from gamma to radio waves travel at the speed of light (about 300,000,000 m/s).

4. Infrared radiation is used to sterilise food and to kill cancer cells.
5. Darker skins absorb more UV light, so less ultraviolet radiation reaches the deeper tissues.

A) 1 and 2   B) 1 and 3   C) 1, 3 and 5   D) 2 and 3   E) 2 and 4

Question 17:

Two carriages of a train collide and then start moving together in the same direction. Carriage 1 has mass 12,000 kg and moves at 5ms^{-1} before the collision. Carriage 2 has mass 8,000 kg and is stationary before the collision. What is the velocity of the two carriages after the collision?

A) 2 ms^{-1} B) 3 ms^{-1} C) 4 ms^{-1} D) 4.5 ms^{-1} E) 5 ms^{-1}

Question 18:

Which of the following statements are true?

1. Control rods are used to absorb electrons in a nuclear reactor to control the chain reaction.
2. Nuclear fusion is commonly used as an energy source.
3. An alpha particle is comprised of two protons and two neutrons and is the same as a helium nucleus.
4. When $^{14}_{6}$C undergoes beta decay, an electron and $^{14}_{7}$N are produced.
5. Beta particles are less ionising than gamma rays and more ionising than alpha particles.

A) 1 and 2
B) 1 and 3
C) 3 and 4

D) 3, 4 and 5
E) None of the statements are true

Question 19:

Simplify fully: $\dfrac{(3x^{\frac{1}{2}})^3}{3x^2}$

A) $\dfrac{3x}{\sqrt{x}}$

B) $\dfrac{9}{x}$

C) $3x^{\frac{1}{2}}$
D) $3x\sqrt{x}$

E) $\dfrac{9}{\sqrt{x}}$

Question 20:

Which of the following are true?

1. Lightning, as well as nitrogen-fixing bacteria, converts nitrogen gas to nitrate compounds.
2. Decomposers return nitrogen to the soil as ammonia.
3. The shells of marine animals contain calcium carbonate, which is derived from dietary carbon.
4. Nitrogen is used to make the amino acids found in proteins.

A) 1 only
B) 1 and 2
C) 2 and 3

D) 2, 3 and 4
E) They are all true

Question 21:

Write $\dfrac{\sqrt{20} - 2}{\sqrt{5} + 3}$ in the form: $p\sqrt{5} + q$

A) $2\sqrt{5} - 4$ B) $3\sqrt{5} - 4$ C) $3\sqrt{5} - 5$ D) $4\sqrt{5} - 6$ E) $5\sqrt{5} + 4$

Question 22:

Which of the following statements are false?

1. Simple molecules do not conduct electricity because there are no free electrons and there is no overall charge.
2. The carbon and silicon atoms in silica are arranged in a giant lattice structure and it has a very high melting point.
3. Ionic compounds do not conduct electricity when dissolved in water or when melted because the ions are too far apart.
4. Alloys are harder than pure metals.

A) 1 and 2   B) 1, 2 and 4   C) 1, 2, 3 and 4   D) 2 and 4   E) 3 only

Question 23:

The graph below shows a circle with radius 5 and centre (0,0).

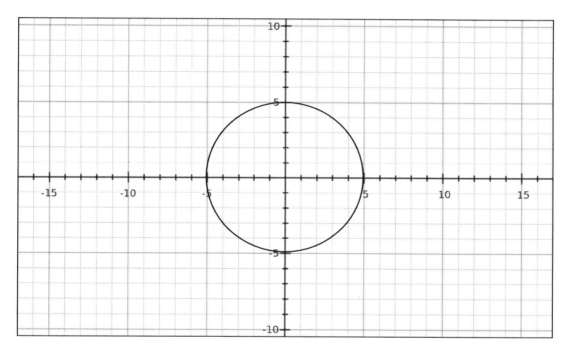

What are the values of x when the line y=3x-5 meets the circle?

A) x=0 or x=3   D) x=1.5 or x=-3
B) x=0 or x=3.5   E) x=1.5 or x=-2
C) x=1 or x=3.5

Question 24:

Which if the following statements regarding heat transfer are correct?

1. Heat energy is transferred from hotter to colder places by conduction because particles in liquid and gases move more quickly when heated.
2. Liquid and gas particles in hot areas are less dense than in cold areas.
3. Radiation does not need particles to travel.
4. Dull surfaces are good at absorbing and poor at reflecting infrared radiation, whereas shiny surfaces are poor at absorbing, but good at reflecting infrared radiation.

A) 1 and 2   A. 1, 2 and 4   B. 2 and 3   C. 2 and 4   D. 4 only

Question 25:
The following points refer to the halogens:

1. Iodine is a grey solid and can be used to sterilise wounds. It forms a purple vapour when warmed.
2. The melting and boiling points increase as you go up the group.
3. Fluorine is very dangerous and reacts instantly with iron wool, whereas iodine must be strongly heated as well as the iron wool for a reaction to occur and the reaction is slow.
4. When bromine is added to sodium chloride, the bromine displaces chlorine from sodium chloride.
5. The hydrogen atom and chlorine atom in hydrogen chloride are joined by a covalent bond.

Which of the above statements are false?

A) 1, 3 and 5   B) 1, 2 and 3   C) 2 and 4   D) 3 only   E) 3, 4 and 5

Question 26:
Consider the triangle right where BE=4cm, EC=2cm and AC=9cm.

What is the length of side DE?

A) 4cm   C) 6cm   E) 8cm
B) 5.5cm   D) 7.5cm

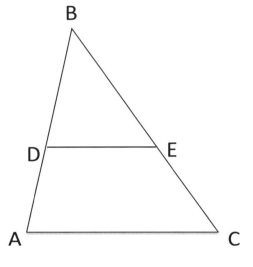

Question 27:
A ball is projected vertically upwards with an initial speed of 40 ms^{-1}. What is the maximum height reached? (Take gravity to be 10 ms^{-2} and assume negligible air resistance).

A) 25m   B) 45m   C) 60m   D) 75m   E) 80m

END OF SECTION

Section 3

1) 'The NHS should not treat obese patients'

Explain what this statement means. Argue to the contrary, that we **should** treat obese patients. To what extent do you agree with this statement?

2) 'We should all become vegetarian'

Explain what this statement means. Argue to the contrary, that we **should not** all become vegetarian. To what extent do you agree with this statement?

3) 'Certain vaccines should be mandatory'

Explain what this statement means. Argue to the contrary, that vaccines **should not** be mandatory. To what extent do you agree with this statement?

4) 'Compassion is the most important quality of a healthcare professional'

Explain what this statement means. Argue to the contrary, that there are more important qualities than compassion for health professionals. To what extent do you agree with this statement?

END OF PAPER

MOCK PAPER D

Section 1

Question 1:
"Competitors need to be able to run 200 metres in under 25 seconds to qualify for a tournament. James, Steven and Joe are attempting to qualify. Steven and Joe run faster than James. James' best time over 200 metres is 26.2 seconds." Which response is definitely true?

A) Only Joe qualifies.

B) James does not qualify.

C) Joe and Steven both qualify.

D) Joe qualifies.

E) No one qualifies.

Question 2:
You spend £5.60 in total on a sandwich, a packet of crisps and a watermelon. The watermelon cost twice as much as the sandwich, and the sandwich cost twice the price of the crisps.
How much did the watermelon cost?

A) £1.20   B) £2.60   C) £2.80   D) £3.20   E) £3.60

Question 3:
Jane, Chloe and Sam are all going by train to a football match. Chloe gets the 2:15pm train. Sam's journey takes twice as long Jane's. Sam catches the 3:00pm train. Jane leaves 20 minutes after Chloe and arrives at 3:25pm. When will Sam arrive?

A) 3:50pm   B) 4:10pm   C) 4:15pm   D) 4:30pm   E) 4:40pm

Question 4:
Michael has eleven sweets. He gives three sweets to Hannah. Hannah now has twice the number of sweets Michael has remaining. How many sweets did Hannah have before the transaction?

A) 11   B) 12   C) 13   D) 14   E) 15

Question 5:
Alex gets a pay rise of 5% plus an extra £6 per week. The flat rate of income tax on his salary is decreased from 14% to 12% at the same time. Alex's old weekly take-home pay after tax is £250 per week.
What will his new weekly take-home pay be, to the nearest whole pound?

A) £260   B) £267   C) £273   D) £279   E) £285

Question 6:
You have four boxes, each containing two cubes. Box A contains two white cubes, Box B contains two black cubes, and Boxes C and D both contain one white cube and one black cube. You pick a box at random and take out one cube. It is a white cube. You then draw another cube from the same box.
What is the probability that this cube is not white?

A) ½   B) ⅓   C) ⅔   D) ¼   E) ¾

Question 7:

Anderson & Co. hire out heavy plant machinery at a cost of £500 per day. There is a surcharge for heavy usage, at a rate of £10 per minute of usage over 80 minutes. Concordia & Co. charge £600 per day for similar machinery, plus £5 for every minute of usage. For what duration of usage are the costs the same for both companies?

A) 100 minutes
B) 130 minutes
C) 140 minutes
D) 170 minutes
E) 180 minutes

Question 8:

Simon is discussing with Seth whether or not a candidate is suitable for a job. When pressed for a weakness at interview, the candidate told Simon that he is a slow eater. Simon argues that this will reduce the candidate's productivity, since he will be inclined to take longer lunch breaks.

Which statement **best** supports Simon's argument?
A) Slow eaters will take longer to eat lunch
B) Longer lunch breaks are a distraction
C) Eating more slowly will reduce the time available to work
D) Eating slowly is a weakness
E) Eating slowly will lead to less time to work efficiently

Question 9:

Three pieces of music are on repeat in different rooms of a house. One piece of music is three minutes long, one is four minutes long and the final one is 100 seconds long. All pieces of music start playing at exactly the same time. How long is it until they are next starting together again?

A) 12 minutes
B) 15 minutes
C) 20 minutes
D) 60 minutes
E) 300 minutes

Question 10:

A car leaves Salisbury at 8:22am and travels 180 miles to Lincoln, arriving at 12:07pm. Near Warwick, the driver stopped for a 14 minute break.
What was its average speed, whilst travelling, in kilometres per hour? It should be assumed that the conversion from miles to kilometres is 1:1.6.

A) 51kph
B) 67kph
C) 77kph
D) 82kph
E) 86kph

Questions 11 and 12 refer to the following data:

Five respondents were asked to estimate the value of three bottles of wine, in pounds sterling.

Respondent	Wine 1	Wine 2	Wine 3
1	13	16	25
2	17	16	23
3	11	17	21
4	13	15	14
5	15	19	29
Actual retail value	8	25	23

Question 11:
What is the mean error made when guessing the value of wine 1?

A) £4.80   B) £5.60   C) £5.80   D) £6.20   E) £6.40

Question 12:
Which respondent guessed most accurately?

A) Respondent 1   C) Respondent 3   E) Respondent 5
B) Respondent 2   D) Respondent 4

Question 13:
"Recently in Kansas, a number of farm animals have been found killed in the fields. The nature of the injuries is mysterious, but consistent with tales of alien activity. Local people talk of a number of UFO sightings, and claim extra terrestrial responsibility. Official investigations into these claims have dismissed them, offering rational explanations for the reported phenomena. However, these official investigations have failed to deal with the point that, even if the UFO sightings can be explained in rational terms, the injuries on the carcasses of the farm animals cannot be. Extra terrestrial beings must therefore be responsible for these attacks."
Which of the following best expresses the main conclusion of this argument?

A) Sightings of UFOs cannot be explained by rational means
B) Recent attacks must have been carried out by extraterrestrial beings
C) The injuries on the carcasses are not due to normal predators
D) UFO sightings are common in Kansas
E) Official investigations were a cover-up

Question 14:
"To make a cake you must prepare the ingredients and then bake it in the oven. You purchase the required ingredients from the shop, however your oven is broken. Therefore you cannot make a cake."
Which of the following arguments has the same structure?

A) To get a good job, you must have a strong CV then impress the recruiter at interview. Your CV was not as good as other applicants; therefore you didn't get the job.
B) To get to Paris, you must either fly or take the Eurostar. There are flight delays due to dense fog, therefore you must take the Eurostar.
C) To borrow a library book, you must go to the library and show your library card. At the library, you realise you have forgotten your library card. Therefore you cannot borrow a book.
D) To clean a bedroom window, you need a ladder and a hosepipe. Since you don't have the right equipment, you cannot clean the window.
E) Bears eat both fruit and fish. The river is frozen, so the bear cannot eat fish.

Question 15:
"Making model ships requires patience, skill and experience. Patience and skill without experience is common – but often such people give up prematurely, since skill without experience is insufficient to make model ships, and patience can quickly be exhausted."
Which of the following summarises the main argument?

A) Most people lack the skill needed to make model ships
B) Making model ships requires experience
C) The most important thing is to get experience
D) Most people make model ships for a short time but give up due to a lack of skill
E) Successful model ship makers need to have several positive traits

Question 16:

"Joseph has a bag of building blocks of various shapes and colours. Some of the cubic ones are black. Some of the black ones are pyramid shaped. All blue ones are cylindrical. There is a green one of each shape. There are some pink shapes."

Which of the following is definitely **NOT** true?

A) Joseph has pink cylindrical blocks

B) Joseph doesn't have pink cylindrical blocks

C) Joseph has blue cubic blocks

D) Joseph has a green pyramid

E) Joseph doesn't have a black sphere

Question 17:

Sam notes that the time on a normal analogue clock is 1540hrs.

What is the smaller angle between the hands on the clock?

A) 110°   B) 120°   C) 130°   D) 140°   E) 150°

Question 18:

A fair 6-faced die has 2 sides painted red. The die is rolled 3 times.

What is the probability that at least one red side has been rolled?

A) $^{8}/_{27}$ B) $^{19}/_{27}$ C) $^{21}/_{27}$ D) $^{24}/_{27}$ E) 1

Question 19:

"In a particular furniture warehouse, all chairs have four legs. No tables have five legs, nor do any have three. Beds have no less than four legs, but one bed has eight as they must have a multiple of four legs. Sofas have four or six legs. Wardrobes have an even number of legs, and sideboards have and odd number. No other furniture has legs. Brian picks a piece of furniture out, and it has six legs."

What can be deduced about this piece of furniture?

A) It is a table

B) It could be either a wardrobe or a sideboard

C) It must be either a table or a sofa

D) It must be either a table, a sofa or a wardrobe

E) It could be either a bed, a table or a sofa

Question 20:

Two friends live 42 miles away from each other. They walk at 3mph towards each other. One of them has a pet falcon which starts to fly at 18mph as soon as the friends set off. The falcon flies back and forth between the two friends until the friends meet. How many miles does the falcon travel in total?

A) 63   B) 84   C) 114   D) 126   E) 252

Question 21:

"Antibiotic resistance is on the increase. As a result, many antibiotics in our vast armoury are becoming ineffective against common infections. Probably the most significant contributor to this is the use of antibiotics in farming, as this exposes bacteria to antibiotics for no good reason, giving the opportunity for resistance to develop. If this worrying trend continues, we might, in 30 years time, be back in the Victorian situation, where people die from skin or chest infections we consider mild today."

Which of the following best represents the overall conclusion of the passage?

A) Antibiotic resistance is a serious issue

B) Antibiotics use in farming is essential

C) The use of antibiotics in farming could cause us serious harm

D) Victorians used to die from diseases we can treat today

E) Antibiotics can treat skin infections

Question 22:

A complete set of maths equipment includes a pen, a pencil, a geometry set and a pad of paper. Pens cost £1.50, pencils cost 50p, paper pads cost £1 and geometry sets cost £3. Sam, Dave and George each want complete sets, but Mr Browett persuades them to share some items. Sam and Dave agree to share a paper pad and a geometry set. George must have his own pen, but agrees that he and Sam can share a pencil.

What is the total amount spent?

A) £12.00   B) £13.50   C) £16.50   D) £17.50   E) £18.00

Question 23:

The figure below shows 12 individual planks arranged such that 5 squares are made with them.
To make 7 squares in total, which two planks need to be moved?

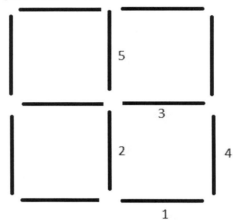

A) 1 and 2   B) 1 and 3   C) 1 and 4   D) 3 and 5   E) 4 and 5

Question 24:

A cube has six sides of different colours. The red side is opposite to black. The blue side is adjacent to white. The purple side is adjacent to blue. The final side is yellow.
Which colour is opposite purple?

A) Red   B) Black   C) Blue   D) White   E) Yellow

Question 25:

UK chocolate businesses purchase 36,000,000kg of cocoa beans each year. Each gram costs the UK 0.3p, from which the supplier takes 20% commission. Of what is left, the local government takes 60% and the distribution company gets 30%.
How much are the cocoa farmers left with per year?

A) £3.68m   B) £6.82m   C) £8.64m   D) £10.8m   E) £11.4m

Question 26:

"Some people with stomach pains and diarrhoea have Giardiasis."
Which of the following statements is supported?
A) Some people have stomach pains, but do not have Giardiasis.
B) Some people with stomach pains and diarrhoea do not have Giardiasis.
C) Kate has Giardiasis. Therefore she has stomach pains.
D) Giardiasis is defined as stomach pains and diarrhoea together.
E) None of the above

Question 27:

Catherine has 6 pairs of red socks, 6 pairs of blue socks and 6 pairs of grey socks in her drawer. Unfortunately, they are not paired together. The light in her room is broken so she cannot see what colour the socks are. She decides to keep taking socks from the drawer until she has a matching pair.

What is the minimum number of socks she needs to take from the drawer to guarantee at least one matching pair can be made?

A) 2   B) 3   C) 4   D) 5   E) 6

Question 28:

Luca and Giovanni are waiters. One month, Luca worked 100 hours at normal pay and 20 hours at overtime pay. Giovanni worked 80 hours at normal pay and 60 hours at overtime pay. Neither received any tips. Luca earned €2000; Giovanni earned €2700.

What is the overtime rate of pay?

A) €10 per hour   C) €20 per hour   E) €30 per hour
B) €15 per hour   D) €25 per hour

Question 29:

"Train A leaves Bristol at 1000hrs and travels at 90mph. Train B leaves Newcastle at 1030hrs and travels at 70mph. The distance between the two cities is 405 miles. Due to a mistake, both trains are travelling on the same track."

Calculate the distance from Bristol, to the nearest whole mile at which the trains will collide.

A) 158 miles   B) 203 miles   C) 228 miles   D) 248 miles   E) 263 miles

Question 30:

"100 pieces of rabbit food will feed one pregnant rabbit and two normal rabbits for a day. 175 pieces of food will feed two pregnant and three normal rabbits for a day. There is no excess food."

Which statement is **FALSE**?
A) A normal rabbit can be fed for longer than a day with 30 pieces of food.
B) 70 pieces of food are sufficient to feed a pregnant rabbit for a day.
C) A pregnant rabbit needs twice as many pieces per day as a normal rabbit.
D) Two pregnant and four normal rabbits will need 200 pieces of food for a day.
E) Three pregnant and ten normal rabbits will need 450 pieces of food for a day.

Question 31:

Michael bought a painting at an auction for £60. After 6 months, he realised the value of the painting had increased, so he sold it for £90. Realising a mistake, he wanted to buy the painting back, which he was able to do for £110. A year later, he then re-sold the painting for £130.

What is Michael's total profit on the painting?

A) £20   B) £30   C) £40   D) £50   E) £60

Question 32:
"Insect pests such as aphids and weevils can be a problem for farmers, as the feed on crops, causing destruction. Thus many farmers spray their crops with pesticides to kill these insects, increasing their crop yield. However, there are also predatory insects such as wasps and beetles that naturally prey on these pests – which are also killed by pesticides. Therefore it would be better to let these natural predators control the pests, rather than by spraying needless chemicals."

Which of the following best describes the flaw in this logic?

A) Many pesticides are expensive, so should not be used unless necessary
B) It fails to consider other problems the pesticides may cause
C) It does not explain why weevils are a problem
D) It fails to assess the effectiveness of natural predators compared to pesticides
E) It does not consider the benefits of using fewer pesticides

Question 33:
A parliament contains 400 members. Last election, there was a majority of 43% of the popular vote to the liberal party. However, as a first-past-the-post system of voting was in effect, they gained 298 seats in parliament.

How many excess members did they have, relative to a straight proportional representation system?

A) 72   B) 98   C) 112   D) 126   E) 148

Question 34:
A cube is painted such that no two faces that touch may be the same colour.

What is the minimum number of colours required for this?

A) 2   B) 3   C) 4   D) 5   E) 6

Question 35:
4 people need to cross a river, one of whom is on a horse. . They make a stable raft, but find it can only take the weight of either two people or the rider alone. The raft must have someone in it to cross the river in order to propel and steer it.

What is the minimum number of journeys the raft must make across the river to get all 4 people to the other side?

A) 3   B) 5   C) 7   D) 9   E) 11

END OF SECTION

Section 2

Question 1:
What role do catalysts fulfil in an exothermic reaction?

A) They reduce the activation energy of the reaction.
B) They decrease the temperature, causing the reaction to occur at a faster rate.
C) They increase the temperature, causing the reaction to occur at a faster rate.
D) They reduce the energy of the reactants in order to trigger the reaction.
E) They increase the activation energy of the reaction.

Question 2:
The pH of a solution has the greatest effect on which type of interaction?

A) Van der Waals
B) Induced dipole
C) Ionic bonding
D) Metallic interaction
E) Hydrogen bonding

Question 3:
How many grams of magnesium chloride are formed when 10 grams of magnesium oxide are dissolved in excess hydrochloric acid? Relative atomic masses: Mg = 24, O = 16, H = 1, Cl = 35.5

A) 10.00
B) 14.95
C) 20.00
D) 23.75
E) 47.55
F) More information needed

Question 4:
A mechanical winch lifts up a bag of grain in a mill from the floor into a hopper.
Assuming that the machine is 100% efficient and lifts the bag vertically only, which of the following statements are **TRUE**?

1. This increases gravitational potential energy
2. The gravitational potential energy is independent of the mass of the grain
3. The work done is the difference between the gravitational potential energy at the hopper and when the grain is on the floor
4. The work done is the difference between the kinetic energy of the grain in the hopper and on the floor

A) 1 only
B) 1 and 3
C) 1 and 4
D) 1, 2 and 3
E) 1, 2 and 4
F) None of the above

Question 5:
A barometer records atmospheric pressure as 10^5 Pa. Recalling that the diameter of the Earth is 1.2×10^7 m, **estimate** the mass of the atmosphere. [Assume g = 10 ms^{-2}, the earth is spherical and that $\pi=3$]

A) 4.5×10^8 kg
B) 4.5×10^{10} kg
C) 4.5×10^{12} kg
D) 4.5×10^{13} kg
E) 4.5×10^{18} kg
F) More information is required

Question 6:
Which of the following in NOT a polymer?

A) Polythene
B) Glycogen
C) Collagen

D) Starch
E) DNA
F) Triglyceride

Question 7:
SIADH is a metabolic disorder caused by an excess of Anti-Diuretic Hormone (ADH) release by the posterior pituitary gland.

Which row best describes the urine produced by a patient with SIADH?

	Volume	Salt Concentration	Glucose
A)	High	Low	Low
B)	High	High	Low
C)	High	High	High
D)	Low	Low	Low
E)	Low	High	Low
F)	Low	High	High

Question 8:
A 6kg missile is fired and decelerates at $6ms^{-2}$.
What is the difference in resistive force compared to a 2kg missile fired and decelerating at $8ms^{-2}$?

A) 8N
B) 12N

C) 16N
D) 20N

E) 24N

Question 9:
Place the following substances in order from most to least reactive:

1 **Sodium**
2 Potassium
3 Aluminium

4 **Zinc**
5 Copper
6 Magnesium

A) 1 » 2 » 6 » 3 » 4 » 5
B) 1 » 2 » 6 » 3 » 5 » 4
C) 2 » 1 » 6 » 3 » 4 » 5

D) 2 » 1 » 6 » 3 » 5 » 4
E) 2 » 6 » 1 » 3 » 4 » 5

Question 10:
The normal cardiac cycle has two phases, systole and diastole.

During diastole, which of the following is **FALSE**?
A) The aortic valve is closed
B) The ventricles are relaxing
C) There is blood in the ventricles

D) The pressure in the aorta increases
E) There is blood in the ventricles

Question 11:

The figure below shows a schematic of a wiring system. All the bulbs have equal resistance. The power supply is 24V.

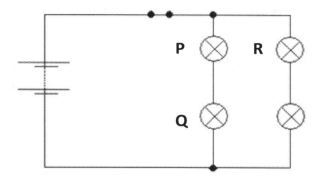

If headlight Q is replaced by a new one with twice the resistance, with the switch closed, which of these combinations of voltage drop across the four bulbs is possible?

	P	Q	R	S
A)	8V	16V	12V	12V
B)	8V	16V	16V	8V
C)	8V	16V	8V	16V
D)	12V	24V	24V	24V
E)	12V	12V	12V	12V
F)	16V	8V	12V	12V
G)	16V	8V	8V	16V
H)	24V	24V	24V	24V
I)	4V	8V	6V	6V
J)	8V	4V	6V	6V

Question 12:

A cup has 144ml of pure deionised water. How many electrons are in the cup due to the water? [Avogadro Constant = 6×10^{23}]

A) 8.64×10^{24}

B) 8.64×10^{25}

C) 1.2×10^{24}

D) 4.8×10^{24}

E) 4.8×10^{25}

Question 13:

Below is a graph showing the concentration of product over time as substrate concentration is increased. Some enzyme inhibitors are introduced.

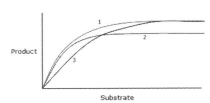

Which, if any, line represents the effect of competitive inhibition?

A) Line 1

B) Line 2

C) Line 3

D) None of these lines

Question 14:

Which of the following is **NOT** present in the plasma membrane?

A) Extrinsic proteins

B) Intrinsic proteins

C) Phospholipids

D) Glycoproteins

E) Nucleic Acids

F) They are all present

Question 15:

There are 1000 international airports in the world. If 4 flights take off every hour from each airport, estimate the annual number of commercial flights worldwide, to the nearest 1 million.

A) 20 million

B) 35 million

C) 37 million

D) 40 million

E) 42 million

F) 44 million

Question 16:

Steve's sports car requires 2.28kg of octane to travel to Pete's house 10 miles away. Calculate the mass of CO_2 produced during the journey.

A) 0.88 kg   B) 1.66 kg   C) 2.64 kg   D) 3.52 kg   E) 5.28 kg   F) 7.04 kg

Question 17:

Given:

$F + G + H = 1$

$F + G - H = 2$

$F - G - H = 3$

Calculate the value of FGH.

A) -2   B) -0.5   C) 0   D) 0.5   E) 2

Question 18:

A pulmonary embolism occurs when a main artery supplying the lungs becomes blocked by a clot that has travelled from somewhere else in the body.

Which option best describes the path of a blood clot that originated in the leg and has caused a pulmonary embolism?

A) Inferior Vena cava   F) Left ventricle
B) Superior Vena cava   G) Pulmonary artery
C) Right atrium   H) Pulmonary vein
D) Right ventricle   I) Aorta
E) Left atrium   J) Coronary artery

A) C, D, H, G   C) I, E, F, G   E) A, C, D, J, G
B) B, C, D, H, G   D) A, C, D, G   F) A, C, D, J, E, F, G

Question 19:

The concentration of chloride in the blood is 100mM. The concentration of thyroxine is 1×10^{-10}kM. Calculate the ratio of thyroxine to chloride ions in the blood.

A) Chloride is 100,000,000 times more concentrated than thyroxine
B) Chloride is 1,000,000 times more concentrated than thyroxine
C) Chloride is 1000 times more concentrated than thyroxine
D) Concentrations of chloride and thyroxine are equal
E) Thyroxine is 1000 times more concentrated than chloride
F) Thyroxine is 1,000,000 times more concentrated than chloride

Question 20:

Put the following types of electromagnetic waves in ascending order of wavelength:

	Shortest -		
		Longest	
A)	Visible Light	Ultraviolet	Infrared	X Ray
B)	Visible Light	Infrared	Ultraviolet	X Ray
C)	Infrared	Visible Light	Ultraviolet	X Ray
D)	Infrared	Visible Light	X Ray	Ultraviolet
E)	X Ray	Ultraviolet	Visible Light	Infrared
F)	X Ray	Ultraviolet	Infrared	Visible Light
G)	Ultraviolet	X Ray	Visible Light	Infrared

Question 21:

How many seconds are there in 66 weeks? [n! = 1 x 2 x 3 x... x n].

A) 7!   B) 8!   C) 9!   D) 10!   E) 11!   F) 12!

Question 22:

Which of the following is **NOT** a hormone?

A) Insulin
B) Glycogen
C) Noradrenaline

D) Cortisol
E) Thyroxine
F) Progesterone

G) None of the above

Question 23:

In a lights display, a 100W water fountain shoots 1L of water vertically upward every second.
What is the maximum height attained by the jet of water, as measured from where it first leaves the fountain?
Assume that there is no air resistance, that the fountain is 100% efficient and g=10 ms^{-2}

A) 2m
B) 5m
C) 10m
D) 20m
E) The initial speed of the jet is required to calculate the maximum height

Question 24:

Which of the following statements regarding neural reflexes is **FALSE**?

A) Reflexes are usually faster than voluntary decisions
B) Reflex actions are faster than endocrine responses
C) The heat-withdrawal reflex is an example of a spinal reflex
D) Reflexes are completely unaffected by the brain
E) Reflexes are present in simple animals
F) Reflexes have both a sensory and motor component

Question 25:

Study the diagram, comprising regular pentagons.
What is the product of **a** and **b**?

A) 580°
B) 1,111°
C) 3,888°

D) 7,420°
E) 9,255°
F) 15552°

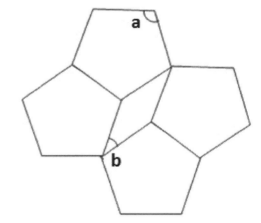

Question 26:

The table below shows the results of a study investigating antibiotic resistance in staphylococcus populations.

Antibiotic	Number of Bacteria tested	Number of Resistant Bacteria
Benzyl-penicillin	10^{11}	98
Chloramphenicol	10^9	1200
Metronidazole	10^8	256
Erythtomycin	10^5	2

A single staphylococcus bacterium is chosen at random from a similar population. Resistance to any one antibiotic is independent of resistance to others.

Calculate the probability that the bacterium selected will be resistant to all four drugs.

A) 1 in 10^{12} B) 1 in 10^6 C) 1 in 10^{20} D) 1 in 10^{25} E) 1 in 10^{30} F) 1 in 10^{35}

Question 27:

Which of the following units is **NOT** a measure of power?

A) W

B) Js^{-1}

C) Nms^{-1}

D) VA

E) $V^2\Omega^{-1}$

F) None of the above.

END OF SECTION

Section 3

1) 'The concept of medical euthanasia is dangerous and should never be permitted within the UK'

Explain the reasoning behind this statement. Suggest an argument against this statement. To what extent, should legislation regarding the prohibition of medical euthanasia in the UK be changed?

2) 'The obstruction of stem-cell research is directly responsible for death arising from stem-cell treatable diseases.'

Explain what this argument means. Argue the contrary. To what extend do you agree with the statement?

3) 'Imagination is more important than knowledge'

Albert Einstein

Explain how this statement could be interpreted in a medical setting. Argue to the contrary that knowledge is more important than imagination in medicine. To what extent do you agree with the statement?

4) "The most important quality of a good doctor is a thorough understanding of science"

Explain what this statement means. Argue in favour of this statement. To what extent do you agree with it?

END OF PAPER

ANSWERS

ANSWER KEY

Paper A				Paper B				Paper C				Paper D			
Section 1		Section 2		Section 1		Section 2		Section 1		Section 2		Section 1		Section 2	
1	C	1	B	1	A	1	D	1	D	1	D	1	B	1	A
2	D	2	D	2	C	2	E	2	D	2	C	2	D	2	E
3	B	3	A	3	C	3	E	3	B	3	C	3	E	3	D
4	D	4	E	4	D	4	E	4	B	4	C	4	C	4	B
5	D	5	D	5	D	5	D	5	B	5	C	5	C	5	E
6	B	6	B	6	B	6	A	6	C	6	E	6	C	6	F
7	A	7	D	7	D	7	A	7	D	7	B	7	E	7	E
8	D	8	E	8	C	8	D	8	D	8	B	8	E	8	D
9	C	9	D	9	B	9	A	9	A	9	A	9	D	9	C
10	E	10	C	10	A	10	D	10	C	10	A	10	D	10	D
11	E	11	B	11	E	11	A	11	D	11	D	11	C	11	A
12	D	12	E	12	D	12	B	12	D	12	D	12	C	12	E
13	E	13	D	13	A	13	C	13	E	13	F	13	B	13	B
14	D	14	C	14	D	14	A	14	A	14	C	14	C	14	E
15	E	15	B	15	E	15	D	15	E	15	E	15	E	15	B
16	A	16	A	16	B	16	D	16	C	16	C	16	C	16	F
17	D	17	E	17	A	17	C	17	E	17	B	17	C	17	D
18	B	18	B	18	B	18	D	18	E	18	C	18	B	18	D
19	C	19	C	19	E	19	D	19	E	19	E	19	D	19	B
20	B	20	A	20	E	20	E	20	C	20	E	20	D	20	E
21	D	21	C	21	D	21	E	21	D	21	A	21	C	21	E
22	E	22	B	22	E	22	E	22	B	22	E	22	B	22	B
23	D	23	C	23	A	23	E	23	D	23	A	23	C	23	C
24	E	24	B	24	B	24	D	24	B	24	D	24	D	24	D
25	B	25	A	25	B	25	D	25	A	25	C	25	C	25	C
26	C	26	B	26	B	26	B	26	A	26	C	26	E	26	D
27	C	27	C	27	D	27	C	27	B	27	E	27	C	27	F
28	B			28	C			28	B			28	D		
29	B			29	B			29	D			29	D		
30	C			30	E			30	C			30	E		
31	C			31	E			31	D			31	D		
32	B			32	C			32	B			32	D		
33	E			33	A			33	E			33	D		
34	D			34	D			34	B			34	B		
35	A			35	D			35	B			35	C		

Raw to Scaled Scores

Section 1								Section 2						
1	1	11	2.8	21	5.4	31	8.3	1	1	11	3.5	21	6.6
2	1	12	3.0	22	5.7	32	8.5	2	1	12	3.7	22	6.9
3	1	13	3.2	23	6.0	33	8.7	3	1.3	13	4	23	7.3
4	1	14	3.5	24	6.3	34	9	4	1.6	14	4.3	24	7.6
5	1.2	15	3.7	25	6.6	35	9	5	1.9	15	4.6	25	8
6	1.5	16	4.0	26	6.9			6	2.2	16	5	26	8.5
7	1.8	17	4.2	27	7.1			7	2.5	17	5.3	27	9
8	2.0	18	4.5	28	7.4			8	2.8	18	5.6		
9	2.3	19	4.8	29	7.7			9	3.0	19	5.9		
10	2.5	20	5.1	30	8.0			10	3.2	20	6.2		

25

MOCK PAPER A ANSWERS

Section 1

Question 1: C

The simplest solution is to calculate the total area at the start as 20 x 20 = 400cm^2. Then recognise that with every fold the area will be reduced by half therefore the area will decrease as follows: 400, 200, 100, 50, 25, 12.5 – requiring a total of 5 folds.

Question 2: D

This is the only correct as it is the only statement that doesn't categorically state a fact that was discussed in conditional tense in the paragraph.

Question 3: B

Off the 50% carrying the parasite 20% are symptomatic. Therefore 0.5 x 0.2 = 10% of the total population are infected and symptomatic. Of which 0.1 x 0.9 = 9% are male.

Question 4: D

The most important part of the question to note is the figure of 30% reduction during sale time. Although A and B are possible the question asks specifically with regard to cost. Therefore, it is only worth waiting for the sale period if the sterling to euro exchange rate does not depreciate more than the magnitude of the sale. As such solution D is the only correct answer as it describes anticipating a loss in sterling value less than 30% against the euro.

Question 5: D

Begin by calculating the number of childminders that can be hired for a 24-hour period as 24 x 8.5 = 204. Therefore, a total of 4 childminders can be hired continually for 24 hours with £184 left over – as the question states the hire has to be for a whole 24-hour period and therefore the remainder £184 cannot be used. As such D is the correct answer of 4 x 4 = 16.

Question 6: B

The simplest way to approach this question is to recognise that there is a difference of £1.50 between peak and off-peak prices for all individuals except students. The total savings can therefore be calculated as (3 + 5 + 1) x 1.5 = 9 x 1.5 = 13.5.

Question 7: A

Karen is a musician, so she must play an instrument, but we do not know how many instruments she plays. Although all oboe players are musicians, it does not mean all musician play the oboe. Similarly, oboes and pianos are instruments, but they are not the only instruments. So, statements b and c are incorrect. Karen is a musician but that merely means that she plays an instrument, we do not know if it is the oboe. So, statement d is incorrect.

Question 8: D

Answers A and B are simply incorrect as the measurement taken is a percentage increase (/decrease) which will normalise baseline diameters therefore allowing for comparison over multiple time points. You should be aware from your studies that ultrasound is an invaluable technique in distinguishing between adjacent tissue types. Any methodology is repeatable if it is correctly chronicled and followed therefore leaving the correct answer of D.

Question 9: C

If both the flight and travel from the airport are delayed this will be the longest the journey could possible take – producing a total journey time of $20 + 15 + 150 + 20 + 25 = 230$ minutes or 3 hours 50 minutes. Therefore given all possible eventualities, to arrive at 5pm, boarding should begin at 13.10pm. Answer D is incorrect as a delayed plan would add 20 minutes to the journey whilst the transport to the meeting at the other end takes a minimum of 15 minutes – even if Megan could teleport instantaneously from the airport to the meeting she would be 5 minutes later than if there wasn't a plane delay.

Question 10: E

This is almost a trick question and simply an application of exponential decay. Recall that an exponential decay is asymptotic to 0 as no matter how small the volume within the cask becomes, only half of it is ever removed. It could be argued that this process cannot continue once a single molecule of whiskey is left – and when splitting that single molecule in half it is no longer whiskey. However, the question does not ask "how long till all the whiskey is gone" but rather "how many minutes will it take for the entire cask to be emptied" and therefore the process can continue infinitely – even if the only thing left in the cask is a collection of quarks … or half that.

Question 11: E

With these questions it is important to only consider information displayed in the graph and not involve any assumptions provided by your prior knowledge. Therefore, this question is questioning your ability to consider correlation as opposed to causation. The graph simply shows that waist size and BMI are positively correlated with one another and that is it. The nature of a scatter plot does not allow you to deduce which of the variables (if any) drives the result observed in the dependent variable. However, the fact that they are correlated is an important result and therefore D is also incorrect.

Question 12: D

A sky view of the arrangement leads to:

C	A	B			A	C	B
D		E	*or*			D	E

In both, D is to the left of E, thus is the only correct answer.

Question 13: E

The question can be expressed as $(40 \times 30) - x(50 \times 30) = 200 = 1,200 - x1,500$. Therefore $x = 2/3$.

Question 14: D

The information given is very much a red herring in this question. This can be solved using your own application of sequence theory. If a sequence is 6 numbers long, the 6 numbers can be re-arranged into a total of 6! possible sequences $= 1 \times 2 \times 3 \times 4 \times 5 \times 6 = 720$

Question 15: E

Although this is an extremely abstract question, all the information needed to answer it is provided. The key rule to have isolated from the information is that with each progressive sequence, a bell can only move one position at most. Therefore, looking through each in turn – for example we can exclude A as the 3 goes from position 4 to position 2. This leaves the only correct answer of B. Recall that the information states bells can only move a maximum of one place – they can of course move 0 places.

Question 16: A

As the largest digit on the number pad is 9, even if 9 was pressed for an infinitely long time the entered code would still average out at no larger than 9. Therefore, it would be impossible to achieve a reference number larger than 9. Indeed, this is an extremely insecure safe but not for the reason described in B (for if the same incorrect number was pressed indefinitely it would never average out as the correct one) but rather because the safe could in theory be opened with a single digit.

Question 17: D

A is incorrect as it ignores the section of the text that states the evolution of resistant strains is driven by the presence of antibiotics themselves. The text states that the rate of bacterial reproduction is a large contributing factor and therefore not wholly responsible – hence B is incorrect. Since this is just one example (and only the information in the text should be considered for these questions) for C to make such a general statement is complete unjustified.

Question 18: B

The fastest way to solve this question is to calculate the quantity of cheese per portion as 200/10 = 20. Which for 350 people would require 350 x 20 = 7000g or 7kg.

Question 19: C

Calculate the calorific content of 12 portions as 12 x 300 = 3,600kcal. As this represents 120%, evaluate what the initial amount would be as (3,600/120) x100 = 3,000kcal.

Question 20: B

Begin by calculating the initial weight of all the ingredients in the Bolognese sauce which comes to a total of 3.05kg. Therefore when cooking for 10 people 3.05 x 4 = 12.2kg of pasta should be used. Which in turn means for 30 people 3 x 12.2 = 36.6kg should be used.

Question 21: D

Calculate the new weight of ingredients in the Bolognese sauce excluding garlic and pancetta which produces a total of 2.8kg. Note that onions represent 0.3kg per 10 people and as such the ratio can be represented as 0.3/2.8 or alternatively dividing top and bottom by 0.3 → 1/9.3

Question 22: E

Begin with calculating total preparation time as 25 x 4 = 100 mins. The fact that Simon can only cook 8 portions at a time is somewhat a red herring as it doesn't impact the calculation. Total cooking time can be calculated as a further 25 x 8 = 200 mins. Producing a total time of 300mins or 5 hours.

Question 23: D

Due to the quantities colour t-shirts are priced at £5 and black and white at £2.50. Therefore, the order will incur a total cost of 50 + (50 x 5) + (200 x 2.5) = £800.

Question 24: E

Answers A and B directly conflict with information presented in the text whilst C and D may well be true but there is insufficient information in the text to address these points. This is an important reminder that although you may well have been a scout and be able to comment on options C and D, you may only consider these arguments in terms of the text provided.

Question 25: B

There are two directions: clockwise and anticlockwise and rats will only collide if they pick opposing directions.
Rat A - clockwise, Rat B - clockwise, Rat C - clockwise = 0.5 x 0.5 x 0.5 = 0.125.
Rat A - anticlockwise, Rat B - anticlockwise, Rat C - anticlockwise = 0.5 x 0.5 x 0.5 = 0.125.
0.125 + 0.125 = 0.25. So, the probability they do not collide is 0.25.

Question 26: C

The article seen here is a particularly good effort at a discursive text as it is completely impartial. Note that the article simply states the facts from either side in equal measure. Nowhere does the author present their opinion on the matter nor do they insinuate their beliefs in anyway.

Question 27: C

The journey time is rounded to the nearest hour (13). Therefore, the longest it could possibly be is 13 hours 29 minutes or it would be round up to 8 hours. Therefore, the latest the ferry will arrive, assuming the travel time estimate is accurate, is given as 20.29.

Question 28: B

The correct answer is 28. Assume, although very unlikely, that you roll a 2 every single go – you will never need to take a step back, only your two forward. Therefore, rolling a lower number in this case is beneficial.

Question 29: B

The simplest way to calculate this is to find the lowest common multiple of the given laptops which is 40 x 60 x 70 = 168,000 seconds = 2,800 minutes = 46.67 hours – although they will not all be on the same lap number at this time.

Question 30: C

A large amount of subtly different data is described here. Of note is the first experiment which describes how nerve conduction is faster in right handed men than it is in left handed men. This result is not transferable to women until it is proven! The experiment currently being conducted only considers dominant hand in men vs. women. That could be either hand or not necessarily the females' right hand. For example, all of the females in this experiment could have been left handed and there is no information in the text to say otherwise, therefore we cannot tell.

Question 31: C

Recognise that two square based pyramids will comprise 8 triangles of base width 5 and height 8; plus, two 5 x 5 squares. Thus, giving at total area of $8(8/2 \times 5) + 2(5 \times 5) = 210$ cm^2

Question 32: B

In order to approach this question first realise that in the first well 1ml of solvent is being combined with 9ml of distilled water producing 1eq of solute in 10ml – hence the first well produces a dilution by a factor of 10. With each progressive dilution the concentration is reduced by a further factor of 10 – hence by well 10 the concentration is at $x/10^{10}$

Question 33: E

The compartments of the human body are occupied by numerous fluids, as the student is only interested in measuring the volume of blood, it is essential he chooses a solute that will only dissolve in blood. So as his known quantity of solute remains no, it must be neither removed nor added during its time in the body. Hence all of the written assumptions must be made and many more.

Question 34: D

The fastest way to approach this question is by calculating the total price per head for the cheapest option as 10 + (8/20) + (10/60) = 10.567. To make the maths simpler this can be rounded safely to £11 a head at this stage. 2,300/11 is approximately equal to 209 which when rounded to the nearest 10 is 210 people.

Question 35: A

Whilst this passage is attempting to weigh up two sides of an argument, it has a clear one-sided approach focussing heavily on the excitement of dangerous sports. It even states that hunting is recognised as exciting by some. Since the previous sentence discussed the link between archery and hunting, the statement is a fair extrapolation to make.

END OF SECTION

Section 2

Question 1: B

Let tail = T, body and legs = B and head = H.

As described in the question H = T + 0.5B and B = T + H.

We have already been told that T = 30Kg.

Therefore, substitute the second equation into the first as H = 30 + 0.5(30 + H).

Re-arranging reveals that -0.5H = 45Kg and therefore the weight of the head is 90Kg, the body and legs 120Kg and as we were told the tail weighs 30Kg.

Thus, giving a total weight of 240Kg

Question 2: D

Recall that kinetic energy can be calculated as $E = 0.5mv^2$. Therefore, if mass remains constant it is the v^2 term that must be reduced to a sixteenth. In other words, $v^2 = 1/16$ and therefore the correct velocity is $1/4x$.

Question 3: A

An organ is defined as comprising multiple tissue types. As blood and skeletal muscle are themselves tissues they cannot be classified as organs.

Question 4: E

This question is best considered in terms of the aerobic respiration equation. With that in mind it becomes apparent that increased forward drive through the reaction will produce large amounts of water and CO_2 whilst demanding an increased supply of O_2. Further from this equation we realise that aerobic respiration produces large amounts of heat, and as such it is expected – in the interest of thermoregulation – that the body will both perspire and vasodilate in attempt to increase heat loss. Therefore, E is the correct answer.

Question 5: D

Recall that the nephron is the smallest functional unit of the kidney. The question therefore is asking you what is the smallest basic functional unit of striated muscle? To which the answer is the sarcomere. Note that a myofibril is a collection of many sarcomeres and is therefore not the correct answer.

Question 6: B

Insulin is a polypeptide hormone released by the pancreas in response to elevated plasma glucose levels. Therefore, it can be expected that plasma glucose concentration will be proportional to the concentration of insulin in the blood. Furthermore, recall that glucagon also released by the pancreas mobilises glucose stores. Therefore, the greatest concentration of plasma glucose would be expected at the time when glucagon is highest during a period of elevated insulin.

Question 7: D

Answers a and c are both nonsense and can be eliminated straight away. You will know from your study of the immune system that it is plasma B cells that produce antibodies and that plasma T cells do not exist. Also recall that an immune response can be mounted as quickly as within a fortnight which leaves the only correct answer d. The passage states that only once blood types are mixed is the immune response initiated, therefore answer d provides an explanation as to how this happens but also why the first-born child is unaffected.

Question 8: E

Haemoglobin is contained within red blood cells and is not free in the blood. Additionally, as a protein it is too large to normally pass through the glomerular filtration barrier. All the other substances are freely filtered.

Question 9: D

An organ consists of many cell types which once differentiated are committed to that single cell line. Therefore, a totipotent stem cell is required to produce the multiple cell types required. In order to ensure that the organ is an exact genetic match, stem cells from the individual in question must be used. Unless that individual is an embryo, adult stem cells must be used.

Question 10: C
You don't need to know the mass of the fish for this one, since there is no acceleration or deceleration taking place. The resistive forces are equivalent to the force of thrust of the fish. Recall that work done = force x distance. Travelling at $2ms^{-1}$, the fish travels 60 seconds x 60 minutes x 2 ms^{-1} = 7200 m in one hour. Therefore the work done against resistive forces is f x d = 2N x 7200 = 14,400J

Question 11: B
The transition metals are the most abundant catalysts – presumably due to their ability to achieve a variable number of stable states. Therefore, the correct answer is the d-block elements.

Question 12: E
Begin by writing down the balanced equation that describes the reaction of francium with water: $2Fr + 2H_2O \rightarrow 2FrOH + H_2$. Next calculate the moles of francium entering the reaction as 1338/223 = 6. We therefore know from the stoichiometry of the equation that this reaction will produce 3 moles of hydrogen. Recall that 1 mole of gas at room temperature and pressure occupies $24dm^3$. Therefore, the hydrogen produced in this reaction will occupy 3 x 24 = $72dm^3$.

Question 13: D
The simplest way to approach this type of question is to assume that there are 10 atoms within the compound. In this case that produces the following result: $C_3H_4F_2Cl$. Next look to see if any of the subscript numbers are divisible by a common factor. Also, if there are any decimals, multiply up by a common factor until only integers are present. In this case the correct answer is achieved straight away.

Question 14: C
This question requires you to have a correct answer from the previous question, although these questions are unfair in the fact that this current question cannot be answered without success in the first part – there are always one or two of these per paper. Simply calculate the Mr of your empirical formula: 113.5. And then divide 340.5 by this: 340.5/113.5 = 3. Therefore, multiply your empirical formula up by a factor of 3.

Question 15: B
The calculation in this question is simple: concentration = mass/volume, what this question is really testing is the manipulation of unorthodox units. Begin by noting the use of g/dL in the final answers and therefore begin by converting the quantities in the question into these units. 1.2 x 10^{10} kg = 1.2 x 10^{13} grams and with 10 decilitres

$$\frac{(1.2 \times 10^{13})}{(4 \times 10^{13})} = 3 \times 10^{-1} \, g/dL.$$

in a litre, 4 x 10^{12} L = 4 x 10^{13} dL.

Question 16: A
A catalyst is not essential for the progression of a chemical reaction, it only acts to lower the activation energy and therefore increase the likelihood and rate of reaction.

Question 17: E
Cationic surfactants represent a class of molecule that demonstrates both hydrophilic and hydrophobic domains. This allows it to act as an emulsifying agent which is particularly useful in the disruption of grease or lipid deposits. Therefore, cationic surfactants have applications in all of the products listed.

Question 18: B
Recall that V = E/Q; therefore, when substituting SI units into these equation it is discovered that V = J/C = JC^{-1}.

Question 19: C
Recall that voltmeters are always connected in parallel – and so that they don't draw any current from the circuit have an infinite resistance. Ammeters on the other hand are connected in series and therefore must not perturb the flow of given, meaning they have zero resistance.

Question 20: A

Much of the information in this question is not needed and is simply put there to distract you. This question can be most quickly solved using the equation F=ma or force = mass x acceleration. As object A is the only things moving in this scenario it is the only source of energy to be considered. Its mass will be the same before and after the collision and so we need only calculate the magnitude of retardation. Given as $(15 - 3)/0.5 = 24ms^{-2}$. Therefore, when plugging into the first equation we realise that F = 12 x 24 = 288N of force dissipated. Alternatively, this question could be solved by calculating the rate of change of momentum.

Question 21: C

Note the atomic masses and numbers in the equation. Whilst the atomic mass has remained constant the atomic number has increased by one and hence the element has changed. The only explanation for this is that a neutron has turned into a proton (and an electron which is represented by x). Therefore, the correct answer is C – beta radioactive decay.

Question 22: B

Begin by calculating the velocity of the wave as speed = wavelength x frequency = 3 x 20 = 60km/s. Which in a time period of one hour (3600s) would equate to a total distance of 60 x 3600 = 216,000km.

Question 23: C

The numerator of the fraction consists of 3 distinct terms or 3 distinct dimensions. As all other functions within the equation are constants one would consider this the volume of a complex 3D shape.

Question 24: B

Expand the larger scientific number so that it reads 10 to the power 6 like so: $4.2 \times 10^{10} = 42000 \times 10^6$. Now that the powers are the same across the numerators, a simple subtraction can be performed $(42000 - 4.2) \times 10^6 = 41995.8 \times 10^6$ which can be simplified to 4.19958×10^{10}. Next consider the division which can be competed in a two-step process, first divide the numerator by 2 like so $(4.19958/2) \times 10^{10} = 2.09979 \times 10^{10}$ and then subtract the powers like so $2.09979 \times 10^{(10-3)} = 2.09979 \times 10^7$.

Question 25: A

Note the triangle formed by the right-angle lines and the tangent. Recall that as this is a right-angle triangle then the other two angles must be 45°. As angles along a straight line add up to 180° a must equal 180 – 45 = 135°. Angles around the origin must add up to 360° and therefore b = (360 – 90)/2 = 135°. Therefore, the correct answer is A.

Question 26: B

The probability of drawing a blue ball (1/21) and then a black ball (1/20) is 1/21 x 1/20 = 1/420. However, note that it is also possible that these balls could also be drawn out in the opposite order. Therefore, the probability must be multiplied by two like so 1/420 x 2 = 2/420 = 1/210.

Question 27: C

The question states that the repeat experiment is identical to the first in all aspects apart from the result. Therefore, although a number of the options may be true like calibration bias, it would have been applied to both experiments and therefore should not affect the result. As such the difference in results is simply due to random chance.

END OF SECTION

Section 3

Doctors should be wearing white coats as it helps produce a placebo effect making the treatment more effective.

➤ This statement addresses the role of the patient's personal experience in his/her cure or treatment of their disease. It is an interesting topic since the role of psychological factors in the treatment of disease is largely unexplored. There is a growing body of evidence that supports the effectiveness of placebo treatments for some diseases when it comes to managing patient symptoms, but there is very little that addresses the role of attire and visual appearance of doctors.

➤ It is also important to immediately question the truth of the statement. There is some evidence to suggest that there is such a thing as a "white coat effect" that influences patient's behaviour and the perception of their problems when they are faced with a doctor. Questioning the statement is very important as it demonstrates that you reflect on the issue.

➤ When answering this question, there are several factors to consider. There is the role that clothing plays in the definition of professions. How does the attire of an individual influence the way he or she is perceived by those receiving his/her service? Some examples here are police officers or judges where the uniforms are heavily tied to the public perception of their profession. Police officers are a particularly good non-medical example since there are uniformed and non-uniformed officers that play different roles playing on the different public perception of uniform and civilian clothing and the fact that without the uniform the police officer is not recognisable. Then the question arises if this should apply for doctors too. Does it make a difference if doctors have clothing that visually separate them from other people in the hospital and does this have an influence on the patient's experience of treatment. Other points to consider when addressing the role of attire is the depiction of doctors in the public sphere. This includes TV shows, books, news etc.

➤ Arguing against the statement is more difficult than it seems simply because you should make sure that you provide a diverse answer that addresses several aspects. On one hand, there is the connection of a specific attire to a specific professional role as described above. On the other hand, there is the question whether attire is relevant to influence the patient's experience to improve health outcome. The whole point of a placebo effect in this context is that it improves the outcome.

➤ Another point to consider when arguing against this statement is the power distribution that comes with the uniforms and whether that is something that is beneficial for the patient-doctor relationship.

➤ Arguing to the contrary, you can look at situations where a professionalization of the doctor-patient relationship can be beneficial. Now, to be clear, the relationship between doctor and patients should always be professional, but in the context of this question, you can use the role of attire and its role in establishing this professionalization. Examples for this include conversations about life-style changes and the role the patient can play in improving his/her own health, especially if this involves giving something up. In this case, attire can give the doctor legitimacy and a certain degree of authority.

"Medicine is a science of uncertainty and an art of probability."

➢ This statement basically addresses the fact that there is no such thing as certainty in medicine. People are different and individual and so is their experience of disease. For this reason, the statement argues that all a doctor can do in terms of approaching a sense of certainty, the doctor should weigh up different probabilities and possibilities of disease. The argument also suggests, that weighing up the different options of diagnoses is an art, rather than acquired knowledge. This suggests some degree of natural talent. It also provides a degree of contrast between the aspect of science that provides the theoretical basis for pretty much every decision we make in medicine and the art of the application of knowledge. It also acknowledges that science always contains a degree of uncertainty, even when individuals believe in the absolute truth of their theory/knowledge.

➢ Arguing to the contrary basically aims at increasing the perceived role of science and certainty versus that of art and uncertainty or flexibility. The main problem with this statement is the general perception associated with the words "science" and art. They naturally lie on different ends of a spectrum with science being associated with facts and certainty and art being associated with softer skills and an absence of certainty.

➢ If you choose to go into a more example oriented direction, there are several points you can raise to write a good and strong essay. One example is the treatment of infectious diseases with antibiotics, especially in severe cases. Often you will find that the disease is treated with a broad-spectrum antibiotic that is likely to target the causative agent based on local experiences and local occurrence of diseases. This is then later adjusted if necessary once a precise identification of the causative agent was possible. Other examples include the stratification of disease causes. One example here is smoking and lung cancer. Whilst it is generally accepted that smoking increases the risk of lung cancer, there are still non-smokers that get lung cancer and life-time smokers that do not. This pattern can be applied to a variety of parameters to result in similar results.

➢ In general, you can keep this essay very philosophical and abstract, or you can aim more at direct examples to illustrate your points. Both options have strengths and weaknesses. A theoretical essay will stay more with the overall style of the statement, whilst a more example oriented essay will be easier to write and to keep track of. However, it will also be more difficult to find appropriate examples.

➢ In the conclusion, when you give your opinion, it pays to be very direct on one hand, but also to be very specific. Depending on which route you took for your main body arguments, this may be easier or more difficult. You can also pick up the idea of medicine being art again as this is an interesting point and ties in with the idea that medicine cannot be exclusively learned from books but should also contain a component of patient interaction.

"The New England Journal of Medicine reports that 9 out of 10 doctors agree that 1 out of 10 doctors is an idiot."

➢ This statement addresses how scientific research will never find complete acceptance in the field. It also suggests that no matter what is being published by even the most highly acclaimed scientific journals, there is always a risk of error. In the end, it illustrates that medical research usually is a game of probabilities as there is never complete certainty when it comes to the pattern of diseases or the optimal treatment of disease.

➢ On a face value level, this question is simple. It is very vague in its assertion, not defining which one of the 10 doctors think that the other is an idiot. Do they all think the same person is an idiot or do they think different persons are idiots? This an important issue to raise when answering this question as it presents a fundamental flaw of the question, especially if one is to apply it to general medical research and research practice. Even in the sometimes uncertain realm of medical research, parameters such as populations of subjects are always clearly defined, which is what gives any form of research value. If this was not the case, research would be completely arbitrary. Coming back to the question then, if all 9 doctors believe that that the one specific one of them is an idiot and they have no prior contact and no connection to each other, then chances are that this single doctor is actually an idiot. If, however, there is no pattern whatsoever to the claim that one doctor is an idiot, then that weakens the claim. Especially if the whole concept is then widened to a population level.

➢ Arguing to the contrary has different obvious points. You can either stay very close to the actual wording of the question which will lead you down a similar road as I have illustrated above, or you can use the question as a parable for the way we conduct scientific research. This will require you to have a good understanding of scientific method.

➢ If you decide to go down the scientific method pathway, you will have several things to point of. Firstly, is the definition of populations, as this is completely ignored in the question. In any form of research defining the pool of data you draw from is essential as only this will deliver accurate and usable information. It is all about reducing vagueness as much as possible. Secondly you need to define the research criteria. What exactly is meant by idiot in this case for example? Only if you formulate a clear-cut goal can you then acquire the data needed to come to a meaningful result. The term 'asking the right questions' comes to mind. Thirdly you need to ensure repeatability. For this you need to define your populations very broadly and in appropriate sizes. You must make sure that there is as little connection between the subjects as possible as this will reduce and bias from personal relationships.

➢ These two options should help you write a strong essay, especially since they can be combined in essentially any way you choose.

"My father was a research scientist in tropical medicine, so I always assumed I would be a scientist, too. I felt that medicine was too vague and inexact, so I chose physics."

➢ There are several components to this question that you need to be aware of if you want to write a good essay. On one hand is the person Stephen Hawking himself. Being a world renowned theoretical physicist, gives the whole quote an almost comical note. This is something you should be aware of as you will always have to point out problems with the questions. Moving beyond this, there are several other points you should be aware of. One is the vagueness of the statement. This obviously is due to the fact that it is taken from what probably was a whole speech, rather than this single passage. Again, something you should point out. Then there is the subject matter of tropical medicine. Tropical medicine is in part still a very new field and a field which much room for exploration simply because there is such a wealth of different life forms in tropical areas that can cause diseases, some of which may never have been observed before. This necessarily adds to the perceived uncertainty. In addition, keep in mind that Stephen Hawking is now 75 years old, which places his father's professional career to the first half of the 20th century, a lot has happened in medicine since then. Secondly you should address the subject matter of physics. Whilst some fields in physics have very little uncertainty and vagueness, a lot of areas are very precise such as gravity or mechanics. So, it is important to make that distinction as physics is such a broad topic.

➢ When it comes to arguing to the contrary, there are several perspectives you can take. On one hand, you can argue that tropical medicine is more accurate than Hawking gives it credit for. An easy way to do this is to enlarge it to general medicine as the clear majority of general medical principles will still apply in tropical medicine, what will change will be different pathogens and the environmental factors influencing pathology and healing processes. If we accept that in general medicine is a fairly exact science, we can use that to support the same claims about tropical medicine.

➢ Another point of attack would be to point out the vagueness of some areas of physics. Easy targets here are String theory and relativity theory. Neither of those can be supported by non-mathematical evidence at this point and even the potential discovery of the Higgs boson in the Cern super collider does not provide enough answers to these questions yet. There are many other examples in the field of physics that are vague, that's why they have given rise to completely separate job description: the theoretical physicist.

➢ Finally, you can also consider Hawking's personal history with medicine. His suffering from ALS for decades and being bound to a wheelchair after far outliving any suggested life-expectancy it is understandable that he considers medicine as somewhat vague. This could well have influenced him in this statement.

END OF PAPER

MOCK PAPER B ANSWERS

Section 1

Question 1: A

If society disagree that vaccinations should be compulsory, then they will not fund them. So, statement A is correct. It attacks the conclusion. Statement b - society does not necessarily mean local so this does not address the argument. Statement c strengthens, not weakens, the argument for vaccinations. Statement d – the wants of healthcare workers do not affect whether vaccinations are necessary.

Question 2: C

Start by calculating the area of wall that may be painted per tin of paint as 10 x 5 = 50m². Therefore, to paint the whole area 1050/50 = 21 tins of paint are required per coat. As such to complete 3 coats it will cost Josh 3 x 21 x 4.99 = 314.37.

Question 3: C

A is a correct assumption as procession is a function of rotational motion. B is a necessary assumption or rather inference of the first sentence. The second sentence only says that an asterism can be used, not that it is the only possible method. Nothing is mentioned of navigating the Southern Hemisphere and therefore C is not a valid assumption.

Question 4: D

Recognise that "bank hours" refers only to hours that the bank is open – which Mon to Fri is 8 hours whereas it is only 6 hours on a Saturday. Although John needs the money by 8pm the bank closes at 5 and that 3 hours difference cannot be used. Hence working backwards John will need 8 hours on the Tuesday, 8 hours on the Monday, Sunday is closed, 6 hours on the Saturday, 8 hours on Friday and 8 hours on Thursday and 4 hours on the Wednesday. With a closing time of 5pm, the latest John can cash the cheque on Wednesday is 1pm.

Question 5: D

First thing to recognise here of course is that individual diamonds can be combined to form larger diamonds with the 5 x 5 diamond the biggest of them all. To avoid counting them all and risking losing count, instead deduced the number of triangles per corner and per side; then multiply up by 4.

Question 6: B

Let my current age = m and my brother's current age = g. The first section of this question can therefore be expressed as m + 4 = 1/3(g + 1) whereas the second half can be represented as 2(m + 20) = g + 20. Therefore, this problem can be solved as simultaneous equations. Rearranged the second equation reads m = 1/2g - 10; when substituted into the first equation we form 1/2g – 10 + 4 = 1/3(g + 1). Expand and simplify to 1/2g – 6 = 1/3g + 1/3 → 1/6g = 6$\frac{1}{3}$ which therefore means my brother's current age = 6$\frac{1}{3}$ / (1/6) = 114/3 = 38. Which means that my current age = 1/2(38) – 10 = 9.

Question 7: D

A is categorically wrong as the first two paragraphs discuss how aneurysms produce inflammation which in turn blunts endothelial NO action. B is incorrect as it states aneurysms directly promote CVD, this is not a direct process. It is the blunted NO which directly produces the CVD. C can be ignored as nowhere are aneurysms categorised like this. E is incorrect as the text states that aneurysms reduce NO which will reduce vasodilatation, thus increasing basal vasoconstriction and thus reducing blood flow. Leaving the correct answer of D which is of course true as observations are not transferable between species until tested scientifically.

Question 8: C

Any statement which refers to national or global figures is instantly incorrect as the text does not mention any statistical analysis has taken place. In order to produce national statistics from a small sample size such as this requires statistical analysis. Whilst E could possibly be true it cannot be stated as there are so many possibilities – perhaps the time of the survey was during rush hour in which case the majority of the traffic would have been travelling in the same direction anyway to reach an industrialised area.

Question 9: B

The runners aren't apart at a constant distance; they get further apart as they run. Xavier and Yolanda are less than 20m apart at the time William finishes. Each runner beats the next runner by the same distance, so they must have the same difference between speeds. When William finishes at 100m and Xavier is at 80m. When Xavier crosses the finish line then Yolanda is at 80m. We need to know where Yolanda is when Xavier is at 80m. William's speed = distance/time = 100/T. Xavier's speed = 80/T. So, Xavier has 80% of William's speed. This makes Yolanda's speed 80% of Xavier's and 64% (80% x 80% = 64%) of William's. So, when William is at 64m when William finishes. 100m - 64m = 36m, thus William beats Yolanda by 36m.

Question 10: A

This question can be solved quickly if you first realise that there is no need to calculate both volumes and subtract the larger from the smaller, instead only convert the television dimensions into metres and then calculate 60% of that.

Question 11: E

From the information provided all the flaws listed are valid since David's main point is that he has chosen the cheapest. A could be true as there is an additional cost of £3 for staying at Whitmore, therefore if the vehicle they are using achieves sufficient miles per gallon then travelling the extra few miles could cost less than £3 in terms of petrol. B again is possible which would argue against it being cheap, as would D. And if C is true then David's argument is flawed altogether.

Question 12: D

C is irrelevant as nowhere does the passage mention standards of modern medical practice. A may be incorrect as nowhere does the article explicitly say that animal testing is the only accepted method of drug approval. B categorically conflicts with the first sentence of the second paragraph.

Question 13: A

Begin by converting all the quantities into terms of items as that is the terminology used on the graph axis. Therefore 12 rugby balls = 6 items and 120 tennis balls = 24 items. Reading from the graph reveals their respective prices as £9 and £5. Therefore, the total cost of products in the order is (6 x 9) + (24 x 5) = 174. Since this is significantly more than £100 the delivery charge is waived.

Question 14: D

Calculate the cost of 10 of everything as (2 x 5) x (10 x 7) x (5 x 9) = £125. Recall that delivery charge is waived at £100 and this therefore a trick question and no delivery charge is applied anyway.

Question 15: E

Tennis balls are sold in the largest pack and so they must be considered. Begin by dividing 1000/5 using the value from the first column = 200. As this is above the range 0 -99 look up the item value in the 100 -499 range where a £1 discount is applied per item. Therefore, in actually fact 1000/4 = 250 items can be purchased which equates to a total of 250 x 5 = 1250 balls.

Question 16: B

Recognise that 120% profit is equivalent to 220% of the original price. In which case the initial purchase price = (1,320/220) x 100 = £600.

Question 17: A
Note that here the question uses the term item and therefore simply read the costs directly off the graph giving a total order cost of (2 x 2000) + (4 x 2000) + (6 x 2000) = 24,000. Recall though that he only pays tax on the amount over £12,000 which in this case is £12,000. Therefore, he pays 12,000/4 = £3,000 tax.

Question 18: B
Lucy must live between Vicky and Shannon. Lucy is Vicky's neighbour, so Shannon cannot have a red door. Vicky lives next to someone with a red door, so Lucy must have the red door. This leaves Shannon with the blue door and Lucy with the white. The green door is across the road and so does not belong to any of them.

Question 19: E

First calculate an average complete one-way journey time as 40 + 5 + 5 = 50 minutes. Deducting his breaks, he works a total of 7 hours 20 or 440 minutes. Since the first train is already loaded his first run will only take 45 minutes leaving 395 minutes to complete his working day. 395/50 = 7 remainder 45. Note that 45 minutes is not enough to fully unload the train, but it is enough to load the train and drive the distance. Therefore, the driver will complete a total of 9 journeys equalling a distance of 198 miles.

Question 20: E
A is not actually a valid assumption as we do not know what proposal conservationists might be bringing to the local councils, they have only expressed their concern. They may well be bringing a proposal to ask for funding to rehome all the species in the affected environment. B is essential to the final paragraph whilst C must be assumed otherwise the councils would not be presenting these proposals at all.

Question 21: D
As there is not really information in the question to calculate the answer quickly. Instead consider each answer in term and calculate the differences to find the correct price difference in the question:
    A)   (3x 1) + (2 x 1.25) – (15 x 0.3) + (10 x 0.5) etc…

Question 22: E
Based on the information in the question options A - D are simply wrong. A is incorrect as antibiotic E has not affected growth at all. B is incorrect as the other antibiotics have significantly affected growth. E was the least effective antibiotic. C was not the most ineffective as it did disrupt growth slightly whereas E had no effect at all. D will now be taken and the experiment repeated with D at numerous concentrations to find the optimum dose.

Question 23: A
1L = 1000 cubic centimetres and therefore the total volume of air Laura needs to produce is 25 x 0.3 = 7.5L.

With a total of 25 balloons she will take 25 x 0.5 = 12.5 seconds breathing in and a further $7.5/4.5 = 1\frac{2}{3}$ minutes inflating the balloons. This yields a total time of 1 minute 40 + 12.5 seconds = 1 minute 52.5 seconds or 112.5 seconds.

Question 24: B
Quickly represent the question schematically as (A = B) $\neq$ (C = D = E). We can now observe that A in fact supports George's argument, C also supports George's argument and D may well be true, but it would have no effect in disrupting the argument, simply only imply D and E are both also equal to 0. However, as E is equal to C it should therefore not equal B.

Question 25: B
This question is much less complicated than it sounds. Begin by just considering a single hour. Throughout the hour of 1 the hour hand will be pointing at 1. Only during the 5th minute of that hour will the minute hand point to the 1 whereas every 5th second of the minute the second-hand points to the 1. All these events will only coincide once. As there are 24 hours in a day 00:00 through to 23:59 this event will happen 24 times.

Question 26: B
A) Potentially correct, but extreme sports also carry higher risks of injury.
B) True.
C) True, but irrelevant for the question.
D) Potentially correct, but irrelevant to the question.

Question 27: D
A) False – we are not told about the healthcare directly but are told that injury and disease posed a threat.
B) False – the terrain was difficult, and mapping was poor.
C) False – outlaws were a significant threat.
D) True – as the text states, there was a marked lack of bridges.

Question 28: C
Whilst B may be true it is not a reason for dependence, only a supporting factor. Dependence implies that we have no choice but to use electricity. Hence A is wrong as gas is readily available; hence D is wrong for the same reason. This leaves the correct answer C which is the only statement which truly describes our absolute necessity for electricity – since electrical appliance by definition only function with electricity.

Question 29: B
First note that 27 guests plus Elin herself means that 28 people will be eating the 3 courses which will require a total of 28 x 3 = 84 glasses of wine. This is a total volume of 84 x 175 = 14.7L = 21 bottles. As wine is only sold in cases of 6, Elin will have to buy 24 bottles so as not to run out. Recall the buy one get one free offer so she only pays for 2 cases.

Question 30: E
Recognise that when rounded to the nearest 10 the shortest an episode could last is 35 minutes. Hence a total of 7 x 12 = 84 episodes would take a total of 84 x 35 = 2,940 minutes = 49 hours.

Question 31: E
Points A and B are the best exemplified through this passage. Often great discoveries come from accidental observations and then exact processes are refined through many experiments in a trial and error fashion until the correct methodology is achieved. The passage demonstrates how as our understanding of the world around us advance so too does our ability to provide healthcare. D can be observed in the passage as the 50/50 split.

Question 32: C
Whilst A and D are true they do not force the stranger to give him the sapphire – remember Jack can be given any stone for a truthful statement. B and C are both lies and will earn Jack nothing. Instead if Jack states E then the stranger has no choice to hand over the sapphire else it would be a false statement.

Question 33: A
Despite the enormous interest rate in Simon's current account it is only awarded twice, whereas in the saver account it is awarded 4 times. Hence earnings from the saver account = 100 x 1.5^4 = £506 whereas earnings from the current account would have stood at £361.

Question 34: D
The largest possible key can be obtained were the first two numbers are at a maximum because they are multiplied together → 9 x 9 = 81. Subtract the smallest number to yield 81 – 1 = 80 and again divide by the smallest number which is 1 hence 80 is the largest possible key.

Question 35: D

A) Incorrect. The text clearly states that the exercise routine is resistance training based.

B) False. Both groups contain equal numbers of men and women per the text.

C) False. Both groups are age matched in the range of 20 to 25 years.

D) Correct. As the only difference between the two shakes is the protein content.

END OF SECTION

Section 2

Question 1: D

As the question states that GLUT2 is ATP independent then answer A) active transport is instantly incorrect as it is ATP dependent. Osmosis is applicable only to water molecules and is therefore incorrect. Exocytosis refers to the movement of molecules out of a cell and is therefore incorrect. Simple diffusion is incorrect as the question states that GLUT2 is essential for the process. This leaves the correct answer of facilitated diffusion.

Question 2: E

In order to answer this question you must recall that anaerobic respiration in humans produces only lactate and energy, whilst in yeast the anaerobic respiratory process yields a molecule of ethanol and CO_2 per glucose molecule. Therefore, there will be 0 mol of CO_2 produced in the human cell culture and you need only work out the moles of CO_2 produced by the yeast cell culture to calculate the difference. There is a total of $5.76/0.18 = 32$ mol of glucose, of which half is supplied to the yeast cell culture. With a stoichiometric ratio of 1:1 in the anaerobic respiration equation a total of 16 mol of CO_2 will be produced.

Question 3: E

Firstly, recall that endocytosis is a process of molecular transport into cells that result in vesicular formation. This question requires you to realise the special case of this which is phagocytosis – conducted by white blood cells in the ingestion of pathogens.

Question 4: E

All of the above statements are true of the Calvin cycle with regards to the Krebs cycle. As the main driver of photosynthesis, we know that the Calvin cycle requires both CO_2 and light in order to conduct ATP dependent reactions. As opposed to the Krebs cycle in man however, the Calvin cycle adopts the use of NADPH as the intermediate in electron transport.

Question 5: D

Option D is one of only 2 graphs that demonstrate a quadratic relationship with the peak enzyme activity correctly placed – pepsin from the stomach close to pH 1, and trypsin secreted by the pancreas and therefore alkaline around pH 13. The curves traced in option c however are far too broad over the pH range to represent enzyme activity. As the pH scale is logarithmic, even a change of 1 or 0.5 can be devastating to enzyme activity.

Question 6: A

This question was taken directly from the BMAT syllabus where many examples are listed for different principles. Reading the BMAT syllabus and highlighting these is a very good idea as well as learning the definitions listed.

Question 7: A

Initially the electron configuration of Mg is 2,8,2. In binding to two chlorine atoms it is effectively ionised to Mg^{2+} and it loses two electrons to leave a complete outer shell and thus the correct answer is 2,8.

Question 8: D

The first thing to note in this trace is that the m/z axis has been cut short. From looking up the mass of calcium in the periodic table one would expect to see the x axis centred around 40. However here the trace is only displaying those isotopes with valence 2 ($z = 2$) hence the values are half the size. Therefore (from the periodic table) when dividing the most abundant isotope of chromium by two, $52/2 = 26$, we confirm that the outlier bar on the right is indeed the contaminant. Therefore, to calculate the actual abundance of Mr 40 calcium ignore the chromium like so: $55/95 = 11/19$.

Question 9: A

Begin by converting the total weight of arsenic into grams like so $15 \times 10^6 = 1.5 \times 10^7$. Then divide by the Mr of arsenic which is 75 (2sf) giving 2×10^5. Don't forget that the sample is at worst 80% pure. Therefore, there will be a minimum of $(2 \times 10^5) \times 0.8 = 1.4 \times 10^5$ moles of pure arsenic.

Question 10: D

Recall that average atomic mass is calculated as the sum of (isotope mass x relative abundance). Therefore $28 = (26 \times 0.6) + (30 \times 0.3) + 0.1x$. Rearranging this equation reveals that $0.1x = 3.4$ and that the mystery isotope therefore has an atomic mass of 34.

Question 11: A

First recall that when a group 2 metal is reacted with steam a metal oxide is formed and therefore the following chemical equation can be drawn: $Mg + H_2O_{(g)} \rightarrow MgO + H_2$. Note the stoichiometric ratio which is simply 1. Next calculate that there is $72/24 = 3$ mol of hydrogen produced. Therefore, assuming that there is 3 mol of all other reactants and the reaction is complete one would expect $3 \times 24.3 = 72.9g$ of magnesium and $3 \times 18 = 54g$ of steam. This is indeed the case and therefore the reaction is complete.

Question 12: B

The reducing agent is the species which is itself reduced in this instance from looking at the oxidation states we can see that that species is S^{2-}. As after the reaction has taken place it has an oxidation state of +6 which would require a loss of negative charge i.e. electrons.

Question 13: C

The highly stable bonds between carbon atoms, and between carbon and hydrogen atoms renders alkanes relatively unreactive. This is important to note as it highlights the major difference between alkanes and alkenes.

Question 14: A

Recall that current = charge/time. The question provides both charge and time in the correct units and so the calculation is relatively simple with no unit conversions required. Therefore current $= 5/15 = 1/3 = 0.33A$. As the question states that the balloon has a negative charge it has therefore gained electrons. Given that a current is defined as a net movement of electrons, in this situation the current must be flowing into the balloon.

Question 15: D

Given that Power = IV it can be deduced that $I = P/V$. Recall that power given in Watts is a measure of the energy transferred per second and therefore has the alternative units Js^{-1}. When substituting these units into the power equation re-arranged for Amps it is revealed that $I = (Js^{-1})/V = A$.

Question 16: D

For a transformer that is 100% efficient power in must equal power out, recalling that P=IV. Therefore, the transformer has a power output of $24 \times 10 = 240W$ which is 80% of the initial input. As such the initial power input was $(240/80) \times 100 = 300W$.

Question 17: C

Begin by calculating the energy required to hoist the mass, this is calculated using the potential energy equation: mgh. Energy = mass x g x height $= 20 \times 10 \times 30 = 6000N$. The power output of the motor is calculated as the joules dissipated per second $= 6000/20 = 300W$

Question 18: D

In order to solve this problem recall that activity = decay constant x number of remaining atoms. Therefore, the decay constant can be calculated simply as $0.36/6 = 0.06$.

Question 19: D

Recall that household electricity is available in the UK at 240V. Begin by calculating the wattage that the bulb is receiving as $0.5 \times 240 = 120W$. Given that the energy rating of the bulb is 80W, we can assume that this bulb is only $80/120 = 66\%$ efficient.

Question 20: E

Begin by subtracting the integral from both sides producing $x - \int_{-z}^{z} 9a - 7 = \dfrac{\sqrt{b^3 - 9st}}{13j}$. Next multiply both

sides by 13j and square, rendering $[13j(x - \int_{-z}^{z} 9a - 7)]^2 = b^3 - 9st$. Finally subtract b^3 from both sides and

divide by -9s leaving the correct answer: $\dfrac{[13j(x - \int_{-z}^{z} 9a - 7)]^2 - b^3}{-9s} = t$.

Question 21: E

Blood pressure in the aorta is the highest of any vessel in the body, as blood has just been ejected from the left ventricle to go to the body. The pressure in the left ventricle (and hence the Aorta) is higher than that in the right ventricle (and hence the Pulmonary Artery) because the pressure must be sufficient to pump to the entire body, rather than just the lungs.

Question 22: E

Begin by drawing your line of best fit, remembering not to force it through the origin. Begin fitting the general equation $y = mx + c$ to your line. Calculate the gradient as $\Delta y/\Delta x$ and read the y intercept off your annotated graph.

Question 23: E

In order to start rearranging the fraction begin by adding m to both sides and squaring to yield $4m^2 = \dfrac{9xy^3z^5}{3x^9yz^4}$.
Now it is clear to see that this can be most simply displayed in terms of powers. E is the correct answer.

Question 24: D

Non-normally distributed data doesn't demonstrate a 50-50 split of data points either side of the mean. Therefore, standard data analysis techniques like normal range are inappropriate (as the formula for normal range is mean $\pm$ 1.96SD). Instead the interquartile range is used.

Question 25: D

Random chance is a large issue particularly in medicine. Clinical trials are inherently flawed as they only consider a very small percentage of the population which is far outweighed by the genetic variation demonstrated within the human genome. Therefore, statistics must be used to transform sample data into data representative of the entire population.

Question 26: B

Begin by calculating the speed of the innermost well as the circumference of travel over time = $20 \times 3.14 = 62.8m/s$. Calculate the outermost well speed in the same manner = $40 \times 3.14 = 125.6m/s$. $125.6 - 62.8 = 62.8m/s$ faster.

Question 27: C

The question states that the repeat experiment is identical to the first in all aspects apart from the result. Therefore, although a number of the options may be true like calibration bias, it would have been applied to both experiments and therefore should not affect the result. As such the difference in results is simply due to random chance.

END OF SECTION
Section 3

"Progress is made by trial and failure; the failures are generally a hundred times more numerous than the successes; yet they are usually left unchronicled."

➢ This statement aims at several aspects of science. On one hand, it aims at scientific method. It demonstrates that science itself is based on trial and error and that to come to the right answer we should test theories repeatedly, adjusting them all the time to become more precise and more in keeping with our results. In the end, it is very rare that a theory survives unchanged. It also stresses that the progress of science is slow and laborious as it requires a constant string of trial an error experiments before providing any results. The second component the statement addresses is the way the scientific progress is seen in the public and even amongst scientists. The common perception is that only success counts and if a theory cannot be proven it is a failure. This of course is a problem since every failure provides a new angle to start from on the hunt for success. Failure becomes necessary for success to be possible.

➢ Since this statement basically has two components, when arguing to the contrary, you will have to demonstrate either that failures stand in a different relationship to success or that the reporting of failures is equal to that of successes. Either is going to be difficult as the stamen itself forms a self-fulfilling prophecy. You cannot disprove it, provided it has some truth to it, since you will not find any evidence for it. So, you will have to focus on a more theoretical level to fund support to argue against the quote.

➢ You can argue that failures, being part of research arte always reflected to some extend in the presentation of data in research papers. They will also appear in the analysis components of any piece of research as failures are essential for the progress of research as it narrows the field of possible answers.

➢ Another perspective you can approach this topic from is to separate the failure and the success. Failure of one theory, even if it had been thought to be correct at some point will lead to evolution of a different idea that builds on the conceptual failures of the previous idea. Thereby, one idea facilitates the other and the failing of one concept will directly result in a new concept that then in turn will either remain a success or become a failure at some point down the line.

➢ You can also consider the role failure plays in our society. It is generally seen as a bad thing and as something to be avoided. This of course does also apply to the scientific community. But at the same time, failure can also provide a new stepping stone for future success, provided lessons are learned from the cause of the failure that can then be applied for future projects.

"He who studies medicine without books sails an uncharted sea, but he who studies medicine without patients does not go to sea at all."

➤ This statement aims directly at the connection between science and soft skills when it comes to the practice of medicine. It claims that medicine is more than just a science that can be learned by theories alone but has a large human component that gives the scientific aspect of medicine meaning. Without the application of the theoretical knowledge, the subject studied has no value at all, at least it cannot be called medicine.

➤ When addressing this statement, there are several tension points you should consider. Firstly, there is the uncharted sea. This symbol has several aspects. On one hand, it is threatening and dangerous as the sailor cannot know where difficult streams and lurking rocks are located. On the other hand, it also has a component of excitement and adventure, just think of the old explores Cook and Columbus etc. Secondly the symbol of not sailing at all. In this again, you can use the sailor metaphor to become fully clear on what he means. Imagine a sailor that has excellent navigational skills but lacks the courage to apply them and so wanders to the harbour every day to stare across the sea. All his skill is wasted as he never sets foot on the waves.

➤ In order to argue against this stamen, you should focus on the first part, the sailing an uncharted sea. This is because the second part holds a deep truth that is difficult to disprove. Even when it comes to medical research, you will have to interact with patients that you draw data from for your research. However, it is simple to argue why books play a vital role in medicine. In this case books are synonymous to all forms of theoretical learning.

➤ The main focus here should be that of safety of the patients. Without books it is only a matter of time until the doctor makes a mistake, crashing his proverbial ship on a proverbial sandbank. Since the focus of medical treatment is the improvement of the patient's condition or quality of life, uncertainty and adventurism have no role in this. At this point it is essential to keep the text on a general level, as medical progress does also come from ignoring the common wisdom. Remember the theory of 4 humours from the Middle Ages, if it hadn't been for somebody breaking with this common wisdom and basis of teaching, modern medicine would never have been born...

➤ If you write an essay about this topic, make sure that you have a very clear position that will give you a good basis to argue from. Also make sure you have fully understood the statement. Due to the use of metaphors this can be tricky, but on the other hand, if you have understood the question, you can use similar metaphors and they will tie in nicely with the question. This will then give your whole essay a smoother appearance and make it better to read.

"Medicine is the restoration of discordant elements; sickness is the discord of the elements infused into the living body"

➢ To understand this statement, you have to understand Leonardo da Vinci. Being an Renaissance artist and scientist, artist and architect, he had a very varied background but also lived in the late 15th and early 16th century which will obviously have influenced his perception of medicine. The idea of discordant elements that are infused in the body and that have to be rebalanced is clear evidence of that since it basically rephrases the theory of the 4 humours that was the basis of pretty much all school medicine pretty much up until the 19th century, when pathogens were discovered and described in their properties to cause disease. In general, however, the statement is to be understood in a sense that disease represents a damaging influence on the body, who's default is health, and the job of medicine is to rectify this influence to restore health.

➢ When arguing against this stamen, there are several possible angles of attack. On one hand, there is the historical aspect of the 4 humours mentioned above. This is pretty straight forwards since you can easily demonstrate why da Vinci would be influenced by this theory and how this theory was inherently false. On the other hand, you can attack the idea of corruption through diseases causing influence by a more general discussion of disease patterns. Whilst it is true that infectious diseases are cause by the insertion of pathogens into the healthy organism, there are a vast amount of diseases that are not. One good example are genetic diseases. Especially those that are inherited in a recessive pattern meaning that parent generations must be carriers and therefore be 'corrupted' as well without displaying the actual disease. If you want to go down the mutation route as well, you can point out that not all change causes negative outcomes since mutations form the basis of evolution and thereby the basis of how we as a species came to be.

➢ The second point of attack to argue against da Vinci here is the role of medicine. Whilst it is generally true that the aim of medicine is to cure the patient, sometimes this is either not possible due to a lack of ability of the medical profession, i.e. we just don't have a cure, or it is not desirable since the risk to the patient if undergoing treatment outweighs the risk of the disease or the benefit of treatment. Good examples here are chemotherapy in the frail and elderly. Another example is that of mutations as the motor of evolution as mentioned above.

➢ To the last part of the question, this statement still holds some truth to modern medicine, consider for example cancer that can be caused by poisonous external influences such as smoking or radiation, in this case the treatment will involve on one hand the removal of the negative stimulus, if possible, and on the other hand the treatment of the negative impact this stimulus has left.

"Modern medicine is a negation of health. It isn't organized to serve human health, but only itself, as an institution. It makes more people sick than it heals."

➤ With this statement, some background knowledge can be very helpful. Ivan Illich was a Croatian-Austrian Priest and philosopher that lived during the 20th century. He is generally known for is critic of the institutions of Western culture such as schools or in this case modern medicine. Looking at the statement itself, it is clear, that the basic message is that medicine has no interest in curing humans but rather prolongs their suffering to sell them as much treatment as possible to fund its own interests.

➤ In order to argue against this stamen, it can be helpful to detect components of truth in it that can then be refuted. One point that can be raised in connection to this statement is that of medicalisation. By labelling everything that does not conform 100% with the ideal of health in medical terms produces a population of sick people that then require treatment.

➤ Another point where the statement holds true is in different health care systems such as the one in the US where maintaining a sick status provides continued income to the doctor and the medical professionals involved in treatment. This is less of an issue in publicly funded environment such as the NHS where there is a stricter regulation of resources and therefore less option for artificial prolongation of treatment requirements.

➤ Arguing against the statement is fairly easy, especially when arguing from the perspective of the NHS. In the NHS, healthcare is provided free of charge for residents and there are no direct barriers in place to block access to health care. This in itself proves Illich wrong since it would serve the institution to make health care a luxury item that comes with the associated price tag.

➤ Arguing that the primary duty of the doctor is not to prolong life is more difficult, since two of the ethical pillars of the medical profession call for doctors not to do harm and to act in the patients' best interest, both of which aim at the prolongation of life in the majority of cases. There are some exceptions to the prolonging life idea, and it is probably safest to approach this part of the question from that angle as it will ensure that you stay on the right track and don't end up in a direction you didn't want to go.

➤ Limitations to the idea of prolonging life are pretty much all the cases falling under palliative care where the idea is to remove suffering and providing symptomatic relief rather than curing the dieses causing the symptoms. Common examples here are cancer in the elderly that are not fit enough to undergo chemotherapy or surgery. Other examples are incurable diseases such as inoperable brain tumours etc.

➤ In this question again, it helps very much to have a clear idea of what you think about the issue. It will make it easier to structure your answer appropriately and it will ensure that you don't navigate yourself into uncertain waters which is fairly easy with this topic, especially when the idea of prolonging life or not is being introduced.

END OF PAPER

MOCK PAPER C ANSWERS

Section 1

Question 1: D

There are three different options for staying at the hotel. They could either pay for three single rooms for £180, one single and one double room for £165, or one four-person room for £215.

Subtracting the cleaning cost for one night would leave:
£180-(3x£12) = £144
£165-(2x£12) = £141
£215-£12 = £203

The cheapest option is one single and one double room and they want to stay three nights, giving £141x3 = £423.

Question 2: D

Glass one starts with 16ml squash and 80ml water. Glass two starts with 72ml squash and 24ml water. 48ml is half of 96ml so 8ml squash and 40ml water is transferred to glass two. Glass two now contains (8+72 = 80ml squash) and (24+40 = 64ml water). Glass two now has a total of 144ml and half of this is transferred to glass one. Glass one now has (40+8 = 48ml squash) and (32+40 = 72ml water). Therefore, glass one has 48ml squash and glass two has 40ml squash.

Question 3: B

B is the main conclusion of the argument. Options A and D both contribute reasons to support the main conclusion of the argument that the HPV vaccination should remain in schools. C is a counter argument, which is a reason given in opposition to the main conclusion. Option E represents a general principle behind the main argument.

Question 4: B

The speed of the bus can be calculated using the relationship: Speed $= \dfrac{distance}{time}$
$\dfrac{3\ km}{0.2\ h} = 15$ kmh^{-1}

The bike speed is therefore ($\dfrac{4}{5}$ x 15 = 12 kmh^{-1}). Considering that the bus leaves 2 minutes after the bike, it is now possible to write an expression, where d is the distance travelled when the bus overtakes the bike:

$$\frac{d\ km}{12\ km/h} = \frac{1}{30}\text{ h} + \frac{d\ km}{15\ km/h}$$

This expression can be solved by multiplying each term by (12 kmh^{-1} x 15 kmh^{-1}):
15d km = 6 km +12d km
3d km = 6 km
d = 2 km

Therefore, the bus overtakes the bike after travelling 2 km.

Question 5: B

Firstly, determine who will move up to set one. Terry, Bahara, Lucy and Shiv all have attendance over 95%. Alex, Bahara and Lucy all have an average test mark over 92. Terry, Bahara, Lucy and Shiv all have less than 5% homework handed in late. Therefore, Bahara and Lucy will both move up a set. Secondly, determine who will receive a certificate. Terry, Bahara, Lucy and Shiv have absences below 4%. Alex, Bahara and Lucy have an average test mark over 89. Bahara and Shiv have at least 98% homework handed in on time. Therefore, only Bahara will receive a certificate.

Question 6: C

Firstly, construct two algebraic equations: A-18=B-25 and A=$\frac{5}{6}$ B

Solve these two equations as simultaneous equations by substituting $\frac{5}{6}$ B for A in equation 1:

$\frac{5}{6}$ B-18=B-25

$7=\frac{1}{6}$B

B=42

Put B=42 back into equation 2: A= 42 x $\frac{5}{6}$
A=35

Question 7: D

I need to make 48 scones, which makes up 8 batches.
8 batches would take: 35+ 7(25+10) +25 = 305 minutes

I need to make 32 cupcakes, which makes up 4 batches.
4 batches would take: 15+ (4x20) =95 minutes

I need to make 48 cucumber sandwiches
This would take (8x5) = 40 minutes

Adding 305, 95 and 40 minutes is 440 minutes in total. 440 minutes is equivalent to 7 hours and 20 minutes. Adding 7 hours and 20 minutes to 10:45am leads to 6:05pm so I will be finished at 6:05pm.

Question 8: D

The volume of a pyramid is given by the equation:

v = $\frac{a^2h}{3}$ where v=volume, a=base and h=height

Rearrange to work out the height for each pyramid: h = $\frac{3v}{a^2}$

Pyramid	Base edge (m)	Volume (m³)	Calculation:	Height (m)
1	3	33	$\frac{3x33}{9}$	11
2	4	64	$\frac{3x64}{16}$	12
3	2	8	$\frac{3x8}{4}$	6
4	6	120	$\frac{3x120}{36}$	10
5	2	8	$\frac{3x8}{4}$	6

6	6	120	$\dfrac{3x120}{36}$	10
7	4	64	$\dfrac{3x64}{16}$	12

The tallest pyramid is 12m and the smallest is 6m. Subtracting the height of the tallest pyramid from the height of the smallest pyramid leaves 6m.

Question 9: A
Work out the two wages by substituting the information provided into the formula:
Jessica's wage is: 210 + 42 - 3.2 = 248.8
Samira's wage is: 210 + 78 - 8.8 = 279.2

Subtracting 248.8 from 279.2 leave 30.4 so the difference between their wages is £30.4.

Question 10: C
The main conclusion is C. A and B both represent reasons to support the main conclusion of the argument. Option D represents an assumption that is not stated in the argument but is required to support the main conclusion that research universities should strongly support teaching. Option E is a counter argument that provides a reason to oppose the main argument.

Question 11: D
D is the main conclusion of the argument. A is a general principle of the argument, but the argument is more specific to the use of helmets rather than the wider concept of danger in sport and the responsibilities of the governing bodies to sports players. Options B and C are reasons to support the main conclusion. Option E is an intermediate conclusion, which acts as support for the next stage of the argument and as a reason to support the main conclusion.

Question 12: D
There are 10 passengers on the tube at the final stop. At stop 5 there were twice the number of passengers on the tube so 20 passengers were at stop 5. At stop 4, there were $\dfrac{5}{2}$ times the number of passengers at stop 5 so 50 passengers were present at stop 4. At stop 3, there were $\dfrac{3}{2}$ times the number of passengers at stop 4 so 75 passengers were on the tube. At stop 2, there were $\dfrac{6}{5}$ times the number of passengers at stop 3 so 90 passengers were present at stop 2. Similarly, at stop 1, there were $\dfrac{6}{5}$ times the number of passengers at stop 2 so at the first stop 108 passengers got on the tube.

Question 13: E
➢ Some students born in winter like English, Art and Music
➢ There is not enough information to tell whether some students born in spring like both Biology and Maths.
➢ We don't know what the students born in spring think about Art.
➢ We don't know what the students born in winter think about Biology.
➢ There is not enough information to know whether this is true or not.

Subject	TIME OF BIRTH		
	SPRING	AUTUMN	WINTER
English	Everyone likes	Everyone likes	Everyone likes
Biology	Some like	No one likes	
Art		Everyone likes	Some like

Music		Everyone likes
Maths	Some like	

Question 14: A

The main conclusion is option A that some works of modern art no longer constitute art. B is not an assumption made by the author as the main conclusion does not rely on *all* modern art being ugly to be valid. C is not an assumption because the argument does not rely on artists studying for decades to produce pieces of work that constitute art. This point is simply used to support the main argument. Options D and E are stated in the argument so are not assumptions. A is an assumption because it is required to be true to support the main conclusion but is not explicitly stated in the argument.

Question 15: E
Reducing the price of the sunglasses by 10% is equivalent to multiplying the price by 0.9. the price of the sunglasses is successively reduced by 10% three times and so the price on Monday is 0.9^3 the price of the sunglasses on Friday. 0.9^3 is equal to 0.729 and so the price of the sunglasses on Monday is 72.9% of the price of the sunglasses on Friday.

Question 16: C
It is easier to write out this calculation in the following format:

a b 7 –
  a b
_____

5 6 5

From the above subtraction it is clear that b must be equal to 2 because 7 minus 2 is equal to 5, which is the unit term of the answer. It is now possible to rewrite the calculation with 2 substituted for b:

a 2 7 –
  a 2
_____

5 6 5

From the above calculation it is possible to gauge certain facts. A must be greater than 5 because 1 is carried over to the second term:

a ^{1}2 7 –
  a 2
_____

 5 6 5

It is now clear than a must be equal to 6 because 12 minus 6 is equal to 6, which is the tens value of the answer.

Question 17: E
Look at the flat cube net and note the shapes that are adjacent to each other. Sides that are joining on the net will be beside each other on the formed cube. Work through to deduce option E can be formed from the cube net shown.

Question 18: E
The H shape is comprised of 12 squares. The shape's area of 588 can be divided by 12 to give 49, which is the area of each individual square. The square root of 49 is 7 and so the side length of each individual square is 7cm. The perimeter of the shape is comprised of 26 sides and the length of each side is 7 so the perimeter of the shape is 182cm.

Question 19: E
The information provided about the child needs to be inserted into the BMI formula: BMI=$35 \div 1.2^2$
1.2 squared is equal to 1.44 and it may be easier to work out 3500 divided by 144. The answer needs to be worked out to 3 decimal places for an answer required to 2 decimal places. The answer to 3 decimal places is 24.305 and so the BMI to 2 decimal places is 24.31.

Question 20: C
It is important that the information is inserted into the formula given for calculating the BMR of a woman rather than a man:
BMR= (10 x weight in kg) + (6.25 x height in cm) – (5 x age in years) -161
BMR = (10 x 80) + (6.25 x 170) – (5 x 32) – 161
BMR= 800 + 1062.5 -160 -161

The BMR of the woman in the question is therefore 1541.5 kcal

Question 21: D

This time, the information needs to be inserted into the formula for calculating the BMI of a man:

BMR= (10 x weight in kg) + (6.25 x height in cm) – (5 x age in years) + 5

BMR= (10 x 80) + (6.25 x 170) – (5 x 45) +5

BMR= 800 + 1062.5 -225 +5

The BMR of the man in the question is therefore 1642.5 kcal. The man does little to no exercise each week. It is therefore required to multiply 1642.5 by 1.2, which gives a daily recommended intake of 1971 kcal.

Question 22: B

Slippery Slope describes a series of loosely connected and increasingly worse events that lead to an extreme conclusion. A is not a flaw because the author does not predict a series of undesirable outcomes. C is not a flaw. It is unlikely that correlation has been confused with cause if the American school did not change other aspects of the school day although this is not explicitly stated in the argument. D is not a flaw. A circular argument assumes what it attempts to prove and this is not the case in this argument. E is a counter argument rather than a flaw. B is the flaw in the argument. Just because moving start times later worked in one school in America does not mean that it will work in all other cases.

Question 23: D

Options A and E, if true, would weaken the argument. If the class is more disrupted this will be detrimental to learning, as will less effective teaching. B does not strengthen the main conclusion, which is based on improvement in academic achievement levels rather than activity levels. C does not strengthen the argument as the school curriculum makes no difference to the argument about the science behind teenage brains. If D is true then it suggests that the improvement in grades is a direct effect of the later school starts rather than a mere correlation.

Question 24: B

The main conclusion is that EnergyFirst is expected to expand its customer base at a rate exceeding its competitors in the ensuing months. A does not directly contradict the main argument. It demonstrates a flaw in the argument in that it ignores the fact that other companies may be stronger in other areas and attract customers by other means. However, it does not serve to weaken the main argument. C does not contradict the main conclusion; EnergyFirst could still expand its customer base at the fastest rate even if there is not much competition between energy companies. D would not weaken the argument as it refers to the rate of new customer intake rather than the number of new customers attracted. E, if true, would strengthen the argument because it suggests that visual advertising would attract new customers. B would weaken the main argument because if it were true then investing the most money in advertising would not serve to attract the most customers.

Question 25: A

Option B points out a flaw in the argument, which attributes the healthier circulatory system of vegetarians to diet, but ignores other potential contributory factors to a healthy circulatory system such as exercise. C is not an assumption: the health benefits of a vegetarian and omnivorous diet are not discussed; rather the argument is centred on the negative health ramifications. D is stated in the argument so is not an assumption and option E is a counter argument, not an assumption. Option A is required to support the main conclusion but is not stated in the argument so is an assumption made in the argument.

Question 26: A

First, calculate the number of hours spent flying and waiting. It takes 24 hours in total from Auckland to London, 11.5 hours from London to Calgary and 8 hours from Calgary to Boston. In total this amounts to 43.5 hours of flying and waiting. Boston is 16 hours behind Auckland and so when Sam arrives in Boston it will be 27.5 hours ahead of 10am. The time in Boston will therefore be 13:30 pm.

Question 27: B
This question requires you to find the lowest common multiple. This is the product of the highest power in each prime factor category.
$18 = 3^2 \times 2$
$33 = 3 \times 11$
$27 = 3^3$

Therefore, 3^3, 11 and 2 need to be multiplied together which equals 594 seconds between simultaneous flashes. 5 minutes or 300 seconds needs to be subtracted from 594 in order to find the length of time until the next flash. The time that they will next flash simultaneously is 294 seconds.

Question 28: B
Firstly, calculate the number of students who play each instrument. 21 students play piano, 12 play violin and 3 play saxophone. Point 1 is true because the sum of 21 piano students and 12 violin students is 33, which is 3 more than the total number of students in the class. Therefore, at least 3 students must play both piano and violin. Point 2 is true because only 12 students actually play the violin so there cannot be more than 12 students playing both piano and violin. Point 3 does not have to be true because some of the 9 students that do not play piano may play the violin.

Question 29: D
One way of answering this question is to set out the result after each game:

	Neil	Simon	Lucy
Start	50	50	50
Game 1	100	25	25
Game 2	50	50	50
Game 3	25	25	100
Game 4	12.5	12.5	125
Game 5	6.25	15.625	128.125

After game 5 Lucy has £128.13, however the question is asking how much money Lucy gains. The difference between 128.125 and 50 is 78.13, so Lucy gains £78.13.

Question 30: C
Option A may explain why young drivers are involved in more accidents but does not need to be true for the main conclusion to hold. B would weaken the argument if true as drivers that spend more time driving will have a greater chance of being involved in accidents regardless of age. D is not an assumption, but if true may weaken the argument as it attributes the accidents to unsafe cars rather than unsafe driving. E is irrelevant to the main conclusion: it does not matter whether the young drivers are male or female; arguably steps should still be taken to reduce the number of accidents. Option C represents an assumption that is not stated in the argument but is required to support the main conclusion.

Question 31: D
The total weight of all of the apples is 6 multiplied by 180g, which equals 1080g. The highest value the heaviest apple could take would occur if all of the other 5 apples weighed the same as the lightest apple. 5 multiplied by 167g, the weight of the lightest apple, is 835g. The difference between the weight of all of the apples (1080g) and 835g gives the highest possible weight of the heaviest apple, which is 245g.

Question 32: B

A) True, but not far-reaching enough.

B) Correct answer. Sugar does indeed have an addictive potential as it causes the release of endorphins and the health concerns are well known. This characteristic makes it like alcohol and smoking, and potentially suitable for similar policies.

C) True, but similar to option A) and thus too limited.

D) Potentially true, but also too limited.

Question 33: E

If we make x the number of sheep sold on day 1, it is possible to write an expression for the profit made on both days:

$$2(\tfrac{7}{8} \times 112)x = 112x + 3528$$
$$(98 \times 2x) = 3528 + (112x)$$
$$84x = 3528$$
$$x = 42$$

The number of sheep sold on day 1 was therefore 42. Since twice the number of sheep were sold on day 2 as day 1, then the total number of sheep sold across the two days is equal to 42 multiplied by 3, which is 126 sheep.

Question 34: B

The main conclusion is that we should not wait for proof of climate change

A and D are reasons to support the main conclusion

C is an analogy

E is a counter argument

Question 35: B

The mean is the sum of all of the numbers divided by the number of terms. From the information, we know that the sum of the first 8 numbers divided by 8 is equal to 44 plus the sum of the first 8 numbers all divided by 10. An expression for this can be written like this:

$$\frac{sum\ of\ 8\ numbers}{8} = y = \frac{sum\ of\ 8\ numbers + 44}{10}$$

Two equations can be derived from the above expression:

10y = sum of 8 numbers +44

8y = sum of 8 numbers

If we subtract the second equation from the first, we are left with: 2y=44 → y=22

The value of y and the average of both sets of numbers is therefore 22.

END OF SECTION

Section 2

Question 1: D

Statement 1 is false. Sucrose is a disaccharide formed by the condensation of two monosaccharides (glucose and fructose).

Statement 2 is false. Lactose is a disaccharide formed by condensation of a glucose molecule with a galactose molecule.

Statement 3 is true. Glucose has two isomers: alpha-glucose and beta-glucose.

Statement 4 is true.

Statement 5 is true.

Question 2: C

Statement 1 is true. High temperatures and pH extremes cause a permanent alteration to the highly specific shape of the active site so that the substrate can no longer bind, and the enzyme no longer works.

Statement 2 is false. Amylase is produced in the salivary glands, pancreas, and small intestine.

Statement 3 is true.

Statement 4 is false. Bile is stored in the gall bladder, but it does travel down the bile duct to neutralise hydrochloric acid found in the stomach.

Statement 5 is true. Fructose is sweeter than glucose so smaller amounts can be used in food used in the slimming industry.

Question 3: C

The combining of food with bile and digestive enzymes occurs in the duodenum of the small intestine. In the ileum of the small intestine, the digested food is absorbed into the blood and lymph. The digested food then progresses into the large intestine. In the colon, water is reabsorbed. Faeces are then stored in the rectum and leave the alimentary canal via the anus.

Question 4: C

Statement 1 is true.

Statement 2 is true. For example, the drug curare, a South American plant toxin which is used in arrow poison, stops the nerve impulse from crossing the synapse and causes paralysis and can stop breathing.

Statement 3 is false. The sheath provides insulation for the nerve axon and increases the speed of impulse transmission via saltatory conduction.

Statement 4 is false. The peripheral nervous system includes motor and sensory neurons carrying impulses between receptors, effectors, and the central nervous system. The CNS consists of the spinal cord and the brain.

Statement 5 is true. A reflex arc travels from sensory neuron to relay neuron to motor neuron and is an innate mechanism designed to keep the animal safe. For example, it allows a person to quickly draw their hand away from a flame.

Question 5: C

Statement 1 is true.

Statement 2 is false. The transition metals are both malleable and ductile, they conduct heat and electricity and they form positive ions when reacted with non-metals.

Statement 3 is true. Thermal decomposition is a reaction whereby a substance breaks down into two or more other substances due to heat. When a transition metal carbonate is heated, metal oxide and carbon dioxide are produced. The carbon dioxide can be collected and will turn limewater cloudy.

An example of this reaction is: $CuCO_3 \rightarrow CuO + CO_2$

Statement 4 is false. Transition metal hydroxides are insoluble in water.

Statement 5 is true.

Question 6: E
There are 9 Sulphur atoms on the left so there must be 9 on the right. Therefore, the values of B and C must add to make 9. This can be written as an equation: B+C=9
It is now useful to try to balance the Oxygen atoms: 4A+36 = 10+4B+4C+14
Simplify to give: 12 = 4B+4C-4A
Equation 1 can now be substituted into equation 2 to give: 12 = (4x9)-4A
24 = 4A
A = 6
There are 6 Potassium atoms on the left. This means that there must also be 6 potassium atoms on the right, so B must by 3. As shown in equation 1, B and C add to make 9 so C must be 6.

$\underline{5}$ PhCH$_3$ + $\underline{\boldsymbol{6}}$ KMnO$_4$ + $\underline{\boldsymbol{9}}$ H$_2$SO$_4$ = $\underline{5}$ PhCOOH + $\underline{\boldsymbol{3}}$ K$_2$SO$_4$ + $\underline{\boldsymbol{6}}$ MnSO$_4$ + $\underline{\boldsymbol{14}}$ H$_2$O

Question 7: B
Statement 1 is true. Males have one X chromosome so if the allele is present they will be affected. Females have two X chromosomes so both need to be affected to be red-green colour blind as the condition is recessive
Statement 2 is true because according to the Punnett square below half of the children will have the homozygous recessive tt genotype and so will be non-rollers.

Statement 3 is true because all of the male children will inherit an X chromosome from the mother which will carry the colour-blind allele.

	T	**t**
t	Tt	tt
t	Tt	tt

Question 8: B
Start by multiplying each term by a^x to give: $a(y+x)=x^2+a^2$
Expand the brackets: $ay+a^x=x^2+a^2$
Subtract a^x from both sides: $ay=x^2+a^2-a^x$
Lastly, divide the both sides by a to get: $y = \dfrac{x^2 + a^2 - ax}{a}$

Question 9: A
This question requires the use of the equation: $C = \dfrac{n}{v}$ where C= concentration, n= moles and v=volume
Convert 25cm^3 into litres to get 0.025 litres and plug the values for concentration and volume into the equation
to get the number of moles: $0.1 = \dfrac{n}{0.025}$ so n=0.0025
This question also requires the use of the equation: $n = \dfrac{m}{Mr}$ where m=mass, n=moles and Mr= molecular mass
The molecular mass is the sum of one calcium and two chlorine atoms which is equal to 111gmol^{-1}.
Inserting the molecular mass and number of moles into the above equation can be used to calculate the mass of calcium chloride: $m = 0.0025 \, x \, 111 = 0.28$g

Question 10: A
The gravitational potential energy of the ball at the top of the slope is *mgh*. The kinetic energy of the ball as it travels down the slope is *0.5mv²*. The gravitational potential energy = kinetic energy, therefore:
$$mgh = 0.5mv^2$$
The mass values on either side cancel out to leave:
$$gh = 0.5v^2$$
Thus we can substitute values into the equation:
$$10 \, x \, 5 = 0.5 \, x \, v^2$$
$$50 = 0.5 \, x \, v^2$$
$$50/0.5 = v^2$$

$$\sqrt{100} = v$$
$$10 = v$$

Question 11: D

Statement 1 is false because the pulmonary artery carries deoxygenated blood from the right ventricle to the lungs.

Statement 2 is true. This property of the aorta allows it to carry blood at high pressure and is why it pulsates.

Statement 3 is false because the mitral valve, otherwise known as the bicuspid valve, is between the left atrium and left ventricle.

Statement 4 is true.

Question 12: D

The Ar of Carbon is 12, Hydrogen is 1 and Oxygen is 16. Therefore, 12g of carbon is 1 mole of carbon; 2g of H is 2 moles of hydrogen and 16g of O is 1 mole of oxygen. The empirical formula is therefore CH_2O. The molecular weight is 30 g.mol^{-1}, which goes into 120 g.mol^{-1} exactly 4 times. The empirical formula must therefore be multiplied by 4 to obtain the molecular formula so the molecular formula is $C_4H_8O_4$.

Question 13: F

None of the above, they are all true facts about digestion.

Question 14: C

The numbers can all be written as a fraction over 36:

➤ $0.\overset{.}{3}$ is the same as $\frac{12}{36}$

➤ 0.75 is the same as $\frac{27}{36}$

➤ $\frac{11}{18}$ is the same as $\frac{22}{36}$

➤ $\frac{62}{72}$ is the same as $\frac{31}{36}$

➤ 0.25 is the same as $\frac{9}{36}$

➤ $\frac{7}{7}$ is the same as $\frac{36}{36}$

Ordering them from lowest to highest gives: $\frac{7}{36}$; 0.25; $0.\overset{.}{3}$; $\frac{11}{18}$; 0.75; $\frac{62}{72}$; $\frac{7}{7}$

Therefore, the median value is $\frac{11}{18}$

Question 15: E

This question requires use of the equation: Percentage yield $= \frac{actual\ yeild\ (g)}{predicted\ yield\ (g)}$ x 100.

If all of the benzene was converted to product (100 percent yield) then 20.5g of nitrobenzene would be produced:

13g C_6H_6 x $\frac{1\ mol\ C6H6}{78g\ C6H6}$ x $\frac{123g\ C6H5NO2}{1\ mol\ C6H5NO2}$ = 20.5g $C_6H_5NO_2.$

However, only 16.4g are actually produced. Using the equation, we can now calculate the percentage yield:

$\frac{16.4g}{20.5g}$ x 100 = 80% yield.

Question 16: C

Statement 1 is true.

Statement 2 is false because infrared has a longer wavelength than visible light.

Statement 3 is true.

Statement 4 is false because gamma radiation and not infrared radiation is used to sterilise food and to kill cancer cells.

Statement 5 is true because darker skins contain a higher amount of melanin pigment, which absorbs UV light.

Question 17: B

This question requires the use of the equation:

p=mv where p=momentum, m=mass and v=velocity.

The total momentum before the collision is equal to the sum of the momentum of carriage 1 (12000 x 5) and carriage 2 (8000 x 0), which is 60,000 kg ms^{-1}. Momentum is conserved before and after the collision so the total momentum after the event also equal 60,000 kg ms^{-1}. The carriages now move together so the combined mass is 20,000kg. Using the equation again, the total momentum (60,000 kg ms^{-1}) divided by the total mass (20,000 kg) gives the velocity of the train carriages after the crash, which is equal to 3 ms^{-1}.

Question 18: C

Statement 1 is false. In a nuclear reactor, every uranium nuclei split to release energy and three neutrons. An explosion could occur if all the neutrons are absorbed by further uranium nuclei as the reaction would escalate out of control. Control rods that are made of boron absorb some of the neutrons and control the chain reaction.

Statement 2 is false. Nuclear fusion occurs when a deuterium and tritium nucleus are forced together. The nuclei both carry a positive charge and consequently, very high temperatures and pressures are required to overcome the electrostatic repulsion. These temperatures and pressures are expensive and hard to repeat and so fusion is not currently suitable as a source of energy.

Statement 4 is true. During beta decay, a neutron transforms into a proton and an electron. The proton remains in the nucleus, whereas the electron is emitted and is referred to as a beta particle. The carbon-14 nucleus now has one more proton and one less neutron, so the atomic number increases by 1 and the atomic mass number remains the same.

Statement 5 is false. Beta particles are more ionising than gamma rays and less ionising than alpha particles.

Question 19: E

Firstly, deal with the term in the brackets: $3^3 = 27$

$$(x^{\frac{1}{2}})^3 = x^{1.5}$$

$$(3x^{\frac{1}{2}})^3 = 27x^{1.5}$$

Next, divide by $3x^2$: $\dfrac{27}{3} = 9$

$$\frac{x^{1.5}}{x^2} = x^{-0.5} = \frac{1}{\sqrt{x}}$$

Answer= $\dfrac{9}{\sqrt{x}}$

Question 20: E

Statement 1 is true.

Statement 2 is true. Decomposers in the soil break down urea and the bodies of dead organisms and this results in the production of ammonia in the soil.

Statement 3 is true.

Statement 4 is true.

Question 21: A

Write $\dfrac{\sqrt{20} - 2}{\sqrt{5} + 3}$ in the form $p\sqrt{5} + q$

Firstly, multiply the term by $\dfrac{\sqrt{5} - 3}{\sqrt{5} - 3}$ (ie 1) and write $\sqrt{20}$ as $2\sqrt{5}$

This gives: $\dfrac{10 - 6\sqrt{5} - 2\sqrt{5} + 6}{5 - 9}$

This simplifies to: $\dfrac{16 - 8\sqrt{5}}{-4}$

This simplifies to: $2\sqrt{5} - 4$

Therefore p= 2 and q= -4

Question 22: E
The question is asking for which of the statements are *false*.
Statement 1 is true.
Statement 2 is true.
Statement 3 is false. Ionic compounds do conduct electricity when dissolved in water or when melted because the ions can move and carry current. On the other hand, solid ionic compounds do not conduct electricity.
Statement 4 is true. Alloys contain different sized atoms, making it harder for the layers of atoms to slide over each other.

Question 23: A
The equation for a circle, with centre at the origin and radius r is $x^2 + y^2 = r^2$
The equation of this circle is therefore $x^2 + y^2 = 25$
Solve the problem using simultaneous equations or by drawing the line onto the graph.
$x^2 + (3x-5)^2 = 25$
This simplifies to $10x^2 - 30x = 0$
$10x(x - 3) = 0$
So x=3 or x=0 where the two graphs intersect

Question 24: D
Statement 1 is false. Heat energy is transferred from hotter to colder places by convection.
Statement 2 is true.
Statement 3 is true. Radiation can travel through a vacuum like space.
Statement 4 is false. Shiny surfaces are poor at reflecting and absorbing infrared radiation and dull surfaces are good at absorbing and reflecting infrared radiation.

Question 25: C
Statement 1 is true.
Statement 2 is false. The melting and boiling points increase as you go down the group.
Statement 3 is true.
Statement 4 is false. Chloride is more reactive than bromine, so no displacement reaction occurs.
Statement 5 is true.

Question 26: C
ABC and DBE are similar triangles because all of the angles are equal.
Therefore:
$$\dfrac{BE}{BC} = \dfrac{DE}{AC}$$
This is the case because the side lengths of the small and large triangles are in proportion to each other.
Substitute the side lengths into the expression:
$$\dfrac{4}{6} = \dfrac{DE}{9}$$
DE=6cm

Question 27: E
This question requires the use of the equation:
$v^2 = u^2 + 2ah$ where v=final velocity, u=initial velocity, a=acceleration and h=height

From the information provided in the question, we know that v=0ms^{-1}, u=40ms^{-1} and a=-10ms^{-2}. Inserting these values into the equation gives:

0=1600 + 2(-10h)

The maximum height reached is therefore 80m.

END OF SECTION

Section 3

'The NHS should not treat obese patients'

Explain what this statement means. Argue to the contrary. To what extent do you agree with the statement?

The statement argues that free health care should not be given to patients with a BMI of 30 or more. This essay will consider both perspectives before arriving at a conclusion.

There are several arguments to support the treatment of obesity by the NHS. The first is that it is in accordance with the definition of a disease; namely that is reduces life expectancy, negatively impacts normal body function and can be induced by genetic factors. Obesity often has a genetic basis, for example the melanocortin-4 receptor polymorphism and leptin receptor deficiency, which shift the homeostatic balance towards weight gain and are associated with hyperphagia and obesity. Obesity can also be a major feature of certain syndromes such as Prader-Willi syndrome, Bardet-Biedl syndrome and Cohen syndrome. If obesity is either classified as a disease or is an unavoidable ramification of certain syndromes then surely it should be treated by the NHS just the same as any other disease.

Moreover, if the NHS refuses to treat obese patients, it will become difficult to decide where to draw the line. Should smokers or people who drink alcohol also be denied free health treatment and how many cigarettes or units per week should qualify? Should all obese people be denied free health treatment or just in cases where it is not an unavoidable secondary result of certain syndromes? Obesity is often a consequence of mental illnesses such as depression and it may be hard to differentiate cause from effect.

On the other hand, obesity in certain cases could be considered as a self-induced condition rather than an actual illness. Individuals arguably exercise a degree of free will and are responsible for the amount of calories that they consume and the amount of exercise that they do. There is an argument that obesity is driven by structural changes in the environment and is a mass phenomenon influenced by advertising and propaganda. Perhaps societal changes in the outlook towards healthy living are required to address the obesity problem.

Many NHS organisations already ration surgery for overweight patients and will not for example pay for joint or hip replacements for patients with a BMI of over 30. Surely NHS funds and taxpayers money is better spent on people who make an effort to maintain a good level of health, for instance patients who are subject to largely unpreventable and serious diseases such as certain cancers.

I would suggest that each case should be considered on an individual basis and that obesity treatments should be included on the NHS where they may act to significantly improve the patient's life in the longer term.

'We should all become vegetarian'

Explain what this statement means. Argue to the contrary, that we should not all become vegetarian. To what extent do you agree with this statement?

This statement is saying that everyone should stop eating meat. This essay will consider both perspectives before arriving at a conclusion.

Some animals are raised in poor living conditions. Circumstances can be cramped and due to growth rate maximisation, animals can develop serious joint problems. Pig tails are cut, chickens have their toenails and beaks clipped and cows are dehorned without painkillers. The slaughter process can also be stressful and inhumane. Halal meat is not stunned before the jugular vein is slit and death is not instantaneous. It could be considered unethical to kill animals for food in this way when vegetarian options are available. Moreover, if farmers grew crops in place of livestock, this would generate more food and potentially alleviate world hunger.

Farming meat also has environmental implications. The overgrazing of livestock entails significant deforestation, which destroys natural habitats and endangers wild species. Enteric fermentation generates huge greenhouse gas emissions and ammonia and hydrogen sulphide leach poisonous nitrate into the water.

A vegetarian diet also has notable health benefits. Diets high in animal protein can cause excretion of calcium, oxalate and uric acid, which contribute to the development of kidney stones and gallstones. Vegetarians absorb more calcium: meat has a high renal acid content which the body neutralises with calcium leached from bones, which can weaken them. A diet rich in legumes, nuts and soy proteins can improve glycaemic control in diabetics. Moreover, growing crops instead of farming livestock can reduce antibiotic use and minimise the development of resistance.

However, there are advantages to eating meat. Meat contains healthy saturated fats that enrich the function of the immune and nervous system. Meat is the best source of vitamin B12 required for nervous and digestive system function and is a better source of iron than vegetables (the body absorbs 15-35% of heme iron found in meat compared to only 2-20% of the non-heme iron found in vegetable sources). Most plants do not contain sufficient levels of essential amino acids.

Moreover, a vegetarian diet can actually have negative environmental consequences. For example, some herbicides utilised on genetically modified crops are toxic to wild plants and animals are often killed during harvest. Eating meat could be considered as natural rather than cruel or unethical. Moreover, the problem of world hunger could partly be attributed to economics and distribution as opposed to insufficient amounts of food.

I would argue that it is ethically acceptable to eat meat so long as it is raised in a satisfactory way. It provides important nutrients, especially for growing children. However, it would be better if we reduced the amount of meat we eat in order to reduce the environmental impact of enteric fermentation and deforestation.

'Certain vaccines should be mandatory'

Explain what this statement means. Argue to the contrary. To what extent do you agree with the statement?

Vaccines are antigenic substances derived from the infectious microorganism itself that provide immunity against a disease. The statement argues that some vaccines should be compulsory. This essay will consider both perspectives before arriving at a conclusion.

Vaccines can protect the individuals that receive them against terrible debilitating diseases. Moreover, vaccines can also protect others in the population. If a certain proportion of the population are protected, herd immunity can be achieved. This means that people who cannot be vaccinated, for instance if they are immunocompromised or undergoing chemotherapy, will not contract the disease. Vaccines can also protect later generations. For instance, mothers vaccinated against rubella reduce the chance of their unborn children acquiring birth defects such as loss of vision, heart defects, cataracts and mental disabilities. Some vaccines have completely eradicated diseases for example the last case of Smallpox occurred in Somalia in 1977. Rinderpest, a disease of cattle, has also been eradicated and the instance of Polio has been substantially reduced.

Although many vaccines are available on the NHS and are funded by the taxpayer, they ultimately cost less to administer than the expense involved in time off work to care for a sick child, long term disability care and medical costs.

Nonetheless, vaccines sometime have serious and occasionally fatal consequences. About one in a million children are at risk of anaphylactic shock. The rotavirus vaccination can result in a type of bowel blockage known as intussusception; and the DPT and MMR vaccines have been associated with seizures, coma and permanent brain damage. Some physicians have raised concerns over the ingredients used in vaccinations. For example, thimerosal has been linked to autism, aluminium taken in excess can cause neurological harm and formaldehyde is a carcinogen that can result in coma, convulsions and death.

It could also be argued that the decision to be vaccinated should constitute a personal medical decision and individuals should be allowed to exert freedom of choice. There are also religious objections to vaccinations. For example the Amish object to vaccines and mandatory vaccinations. The Catholic Church is also opposed to the ingredients of certain vaccinations. For example, the MMR vaccine is cultivated in cells derived from two foetuses aborted in the 1960s.

However, the chance of serious side effects is incredibly small and furthermore the ingredients in vaccines are safe in the tiny amounts used: the exposure of children to aluminium is higher in breast milk than it is in vaccines. The FDA (food and drug administration) requires vaccines to be tested for up to 10 years before they are licensed and even after licensing, they continue to be monitored. In my view, the wider benefits of vaccines outweigh the minimal risk of poor side effects. In addition, it could be argued that personal decisions should be restricted when they affect the health of others. Therefore, I am supportive of certain vaccinations being mandatory.

'Compassion is the most important quality of a healthcare professional'

Explain what this statement means. Argue to the contrary. To what extent do you agree with the statement?

The statement argues that in careers involved in caring for the sick; kindness and empathy for the patients is the most important professional attribute. I will provide reasons for why this might be the case, whilst also discussing the importance of a sound scientific knowledge. I will then decide which quality I believe to be the most important.

A lack of compassion in care homes and hospitals could be held partly responsible for inexcusable cases of patient neglect. For example, care home members have been mocked and tortured and in hospitals, patients have been left surrounded in their own urine and forced to drink water from flower vases. Arguably this neglect has arisen from a lack of care and compassion from the healthcare professionals. However, at the same time it must partly be attributed to understaffing, lack of resources and training. Moreover, it is difficult to assess someone's level of compassion and it is uncertain whether this is something that can actually be taught.

A greater level of compassion would lead to better diagnoses. A large aspect of healthcare involves listening and communicating to patients. If a doctor has more empathy, patients are more likely to trust their doctor and disclose more personal information. An empathetic manner has also been shown to reduce patient anxiety and lead to faster patient recovery.

On the other hand, too much empathy could actually hamper healthcare professionals. Doctors and other health workers often require a degree of objectivity in order to make optimal decisions that may go against the patient's wishes. A level of detachment would also help professionals to remain calm in stressful clinical situations. Clearly, it is desirable for doctors and other healthcare professionals to have a detailed and comprehensive medical knowledge contributing to faster diagnoses, more skilled treatments and faster recoveries.

I would argue that scientific knowledge is the most important quality of a doctor especially because it is a necessity in order to practice medicine. However, compassion is also a highly important quality in a healthcare worker and is what separates an adequate doctor or nurse from an exceptional one.

END OF PAPER

MOCK PAPER D ANSWERS

Section 1

Question 1: B
James runs 26.2 seconds, which is outside the qualifying time, therefore he does not qualify.

Question 2: D
Using s as the sandwich price, c for the crisps and w for the watermelon, the equation to solve is
£5.60 $= s + c + w$.
Substituting in the information that $w = 2s$ and $s = 2c$:
£5.60 $= s + 2s + s/2$ or £5.60 $= 3.5\,s$
$s =$ £1.60
$Hence, w = 2 \times £160 = £320$

Question 3: E
Jane leaves at 2:35pm and arrives at 3:25pm, taking 50 minutes. Sam's journey takes twice as long, so leaving at 3:00pm it takes 100 minutes, giving an arrival time of 4:40pm.

Question 4: C
After the transaction, Michael has eight sweets. Therefore Hannah has 16 sweets after the transaction and hence 13 sweets before.

Question 5: C
Find original pay: £250/0.86 = 290 basic original pay. Add the rise: (290 x 1.05) + 6 = £311 new basic pay.
Subtract the income tax at 12% = 311 x 0.88 = £273 new pay rate

Question 6: C
Given the first cube is a white cube, you are drawing from one of three boxes, boxes A, C or D. Boxes C and D will have just had their only white cube removed, whereas box A will have one white cube remaining. Therefore the probability of drawing a second white cube is $^1/_3$, thus the probability of non-white (i.e. black) is $^2/_3$.

Question 7: E
This is a simultaneous equations question.
 500 + 10(x − 80) = 600 + 5x; true when x ≥ 80.
500 + 10x − 800 = 600 + 5x
» 5x = 900
» x = 180, therefore after 180 minutes

Question 8: E
The keyword here is **efficiency**. Simon's argument is that a slow eater will be less productive. Whilst eating slowly might be a weakness (D) and lunch breaks might be considered a distraction (B), they do not directly support Simon's argument.
Although eating slow may lead to longer lunches (A) and reduce the time available to work (C), this doesn't necessarily mean the individual will be less productive – the lunch break might make them more efficient than other individuals. In order for Simon to assume slow eaters will be less productive, it must follow that slower eaters will have less time to work **efficiently** (E).

Question 9: D
This is a LCM question. We need to find the lowest common multiple of the song lengths. The LCM of 100, 180 and 240 is 3,600 seconds – equal to 60 minutes. For ease of arithmetic, you may choose to work reduce all numbers by a factor of 10.

Question 10: D

The journey is 3 hours and 45 mins, minus a 14 minute break gives 3hrs 31 mins travel time, or 211 minutes. Therefore the average speed is 51mph, or 82kmh by using the stated conversion factor.

Question 11: C

The mean guess is £13.80, which is £5.80 too high.

Question 12: C

The overall error for respondent 3 is £13, which is the least.

Question 13; B

The passage suggests that the attacks were carried out by extra terrestrial beings. Though the supposed UFO sightings have rational explanations, the writer feels this is insufficient to dismiss his idea.

Question 14: C

The initial argument suggests that two things must be present for an action to happen. If only one is absent, the action cannot happen. Argument C has the same form, the others do not.

Question 15: E

Building model ships requires several positive traits. The passage does not tell us which is the most important or most commonly lacked skill, only that more than one skill is required for success.

Question 16: C

Joseph does not have blue cubic blocks, since all his blue blocks are cylindrical.

Question 17: C

Each hour is a 1/12 of a complete turn of the clock face, equalling 30°. In an hour, the hour hand rotates 30°, so 10° every 20 minutes. The distance between the numbers 4 and 8 on a clock face is 4 x 30 = 120. There is still 1/3 of the distance between 3 and 4 to go, so you need to add 10° to get the total angle.

Question 18: B

The chance of red is 2/6 = 1/3. To get no reds at all, it must be non-red for each of three independent rolls. The probability of this is $(2/3)^3 = 8/27$. Therefore the probability of at least one red is 1 – 8/27 = 19/27

Question 19: D

These three furniture items are compatible with having 6 legs. All the other statements are false.

Question 20: D

Work this out by time. The friends are closing on each other at a total of 6mph overall, therefore the 42 miles take 7 hours. In seven hours, the falcon, flying at 18mph covers 18 x 7 = 126 miles.

Question 21: C

The passage tells us that antibiotic resistance could lead to people dying from Victorian diseases, and that liberal use of antibiotics in farming is the "most significant" contributor to this. Therefore it would be true to say that this use of antibiotics could cause serious harm.

Question 22: B

Calculate the overall cost of three stationery sets, then subtract any items not bought. For each item shared between two people, there is one of that item not required. The overall cost is £6.00 per person, £18.00 overall. Subtract one geometry set (£3), one paper pad (£1) and one pencil (50p) to give £13.50 overall cost.

Question 23: C

Moving planks 1 and 4 to form a cross inside one of the other squares will solve the problem. Two squares are broken (the bottom right hand corner and the overall large square) but four new small ones are created, bringing the total up to seven.

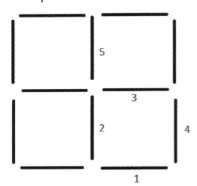
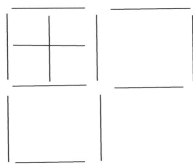

Question 24: D

The purple square is opposite white, since both are adjacent to blue on opposite sides. White and purple cannot be adjacent to each other since the position of the opposite black and red sides makes that impossible.

Question 25: C

We take the overall price to the UK and subtract money which does not go to the farmers. 36,000,000kg at 300p/kg gives £108m. Subtract commission 108 x 0.8, then take 10% of the remaining proceeds as the farmers' share, giving £8.64m

Question 26: E

None of the responses can be reliably deduced from the statement regarding the Giardiasis. It cannot be A, because the statement relates to both stomach pain and diarrhoea. It cannot be B as the statement only refers to individuals with Giardisis – we do not know if people with these symptoms do not have Giardiasis. It cannot be C and D due to the natures of the statement itself.

Question 27: C

Catherine must choose four socks. If choosing three or fewer, it is possible that they could each be of different colour. When choosing four, it is certain that at least two socks will make a matching pair, but possible that there will be two pairs.

Question 28: D

This is another simultaneous equations question. Solve to find x, the normal rate of pay.
$100x + 20y = 2000$ » $60y = 6000 – 300x$ (substitute this into the equation representing Giovanni's pay)
$80x + 60y = 2700$
» $80x + (6000 – 300x) = 2700$
» $220x = 3300$
$x = 15$
To get the value for overtime rate of pay, substitute x back into one of the two equations and solve for y
$100(15) + 20y = 2000$
$Y = 25$
So the overtime rate of pay is 25 euros per hour.

Question 29: E

The easiest way to do this is via simultaneous equations to solve for the time when both trains collide (x). Let A be the distance travelled by the Bristol train and B the distance travelled by the Newcastle train. Using Distance = speed x time. :

A = 90x + 45 (to account for the extra ½ hour which this train has been travelling relative to B, at 90miles an hour) and B = 70x

The collision will occur when the total distance travelled by both trains is = 405

i.e. A + B =405

Therefore, 90x + 45 + 70x = 405

X =2.25 hours. Thus, collision happens at 12:45.

Substitute x=2.25 into the first equation to give the distance from Bristol:

A = 90 x 2.25 + 45 = 247.5

Question 30: E

Form simultaneous equations to do this quickly. Let x be pregnant rabbits and y be non-pregnant rabbits. 100 = x + 2y and 175 = 2x +3y. Substituting for x gives 175 = 2(100-2y) +3y. Solve for y = 25 and therefore x = 50 when substituted back into 100 = x +2y. Only E doesn't concord with these values.

Question 31: D

Michael pays £60 and £110 = £170 for the painting. He sells it for £90 and £130 = £220. Thus, he makes a profit of £220 - £170 = £50.

Question 32: D

The principle problem is that it does not compare the relative effectiveness of pesticides and natural predators. It might be that pesticides are far more effective at controlling pests, despite the unnecessary excess killing.

Question 33: D

Proportionately, there would be 172 members. Therefore there is an excess of 298 – 172 = 126 members.

Question 34: B

If each pair of opposite faces is painted one colour, this requirement can be satisfied with a minimum of three colours.

Question 35: C

Two people cross dropping one (first crossing) on the other side. One returns (second) and then takes another person over (third). When one returns this time (fourth) he leaves two on the correct bank and returns for the rider alone on the wrong side. The rider comes back alone leaving one person on the wrong side (five) and one of the people (six) return to collect the final person. These two return together completing the 7th crossing.

END OF SECTION

Section 2

Question 1: A
This is a straightforward question that tests basic understanding of kinetics. Catalysts help overcome energy barriers by reducing the activation energy necessary for a reaction.

Question 2: E
Recall that pH is a logarithmic scale of proton concentration and therefore will have the largest effect on hydrogen bonding.

Question 3: D
The balanced equation for the reaction between magnesium oxide and hydrochloric acid is:
$MgO + 2HCl \rightarrow MgCl2 + H2$
The relative molecular mass of MgO is $24 + 16 = 40g$ per mole.
Therefore 10g of MgO represents $10/40 = 0.25$ moles.
As the ratio of MgO to MgCl2 is 1:1, we know that the amount of MgCl2 produced will also be 0.25 moles. One mole of MgCl2 has a molecular mass of $24 + (2 \times 35.5) = 95g$ per mole.
Therefore the reaction will produce $0.25 \times 95 = 23.75g$ of MgCl2.

Question 4: B
Gravitational potential energy increases as the grain is lifted further from floor; this is equal to the work done against gravity to attain the higher position. The potential energy equal to $mg\Delta h$, so it is dependent upon the mass of the grain that is lifted.

Question 5: E
This is a tricky question that requires a conceptual leap. Only the top candidates will get this correct.

Surface Area of Earth $= 4\pi r^2$
$= 4 \times 3 \times (0.6 \times 10^7)^2$
$= 12 \times (6 \times 10^6)^2$
$= 12 \times 36 \times 10^{12}$
$= 3.6 \times 10^{14}$

Since $= \dfrac{Force}{Area}$, $Atmospheric\ Pressure = \dfrac{Force\ exerted\ by atmosphere}{Surface\ Area\ of\ Earth}$

Therefore: $Force = 10^5 x\ 3.6 \times 10^{14}$
$= 3.6 \times 10^{19}\ N$

The force exerted by the atmosphere is equal to its weight therefore:
$Force = Weight = mass\ x\ g$

Hence, $Atmospheric\ Mass = \dfrac{3.6 \times 10^{19}}{10} = 3.6 \times 10^{18}\ Kg$

Question 6: F
A polymer consists of repeating monomeric subunits. Polythene consists of multiple ethenes; glycogen of glucose; collagen of amino acids, starch of glucose; DNA of nucleotide bases, but triglycerides are not composed of monomeric subunits.

Question 7: E
Increased ADH causes more water reabsorption. This concentrates the sodium in the urine by reducing urine volume. In the healthy kidney, all glucose is reabsorbed and none is excreted into the urine.

Question 8: D
$F = ma$; therefore the difference in force is equal to $m_1a_1 - m_2a_2$. This equals $(6 \times 6) - (2 \times 8) = 20N$

Question 9: C
It's important to know your reactivity series as its easy marks. Remember that potassium is more reactive than sodium, as it has a greater number of electron shells, with the outermost single electron being more loosely attracted to the nucleus because of this, and hence more likely to be lost. Following this pattern, sodium is the next most reactive and copper the least.

Question 10: D
Diastole is the relaxation phase of the cardiac cycle. In diastole the pressure in the aorta decreases as the contractile force from the ventricles is reduced. All of the other statements are true; the aortic valve closes after ventricular systole. All four chambers of the heart have blood in them throughout the cardiac cycle.

Question 11: A
Because the two sides of the circuit are in parallel, both sets of lights experience a 24v voltage drop across them. In lights R and S this is shared equally between them, but in lights P and Q, the new light with twice the resistance takes twice the voltage in accordance with Ohm's Law ($V = IR$).

Question 12: E
144ml of water is 144g, which is the equivalent of 8 moles. 8 times Avogadro's constant gives the number of molecules present, which is 4.8×10^{24}. There are 10 protons and 10 electrons in each water molecule, hence there are 4.8×10^{25} electrons.

Question 13: B
Competitive inhibition occurs when the inhibitor prevents a reaction by binding to the enzyme active site. Hence, a higher concentration of the substrate can result in the same overall rate of reaction. i.e. the substrate outcompetes the competitor.

Non competitive inhibition is where the inhibitor binds to the enzyme (not at the active site) and prevents the reaction from taking place. Increasing the substrate concentration therefore does not increase the reaction rate i.e. the substrate cannot outcompete the competitor as the enzymes are disabled and the competitor is not binding to the active site.

In this graph, line 1 shows the normal reaction without inhibition, line 2 shows competitive inhibitor and line 3 shows non-competitive inhibition.

Question 14: E
Nucleic acids are only found in the nucleus (DNA & RNA) and cytoplasm (RNA). They are not a component of the plasma membrane, whereas the other molecules are.

Question 15: B
Number of annual flights = Flights per hour x Number of hours in one year x Number of airports
$= 4 \, x \, (24 \, x \, 365) \, x \, 1000$
$= 96 \, x \, 365 \, x \, (1000)$
$\approx 100 \, x \, 365 \, x \, 10 \, x \, 100$
$= 365 \, x \, 10^5 = 36.5 \, Million$

However, this is an overestimate since we have multiplied by 100 instead of 96. Hence, the actual answer will be slightly lower. 35 Million is the only other viable option available.
365x24=8760 is the number of hours in a year, then 8760 x number of flights per hour (4) = 35040 flights per year per airport. Multiply by the number of airports – 42 million to the nearest million.

Question 16: F
Write the equation to calculate molar ratios:
$C_8H_{18} + 12.5\ O_2 \rightarrow 8CO_2 + 9H_2O$
Travelling 10 miles uses: 228 x 10 = 2,280g of Octane.
M_r of Octane = 12 x 8 + 18 x 1 = 114
Number of moles of octane used = 2,280/114 = 20 moles.
Thus, 160 moles of CO_2 must be produced.
M_r of CO_2 = 12 + 16 x 2= 44
Mass of CO_2 produced = 44 x 160
= 7,040 g = 7.04 kg

Question 17: D
Add the first and last equations together to give: 2F = 4, thus F = 2.
Then add the second and third equations to give 2F – 2H= 5. Thus, H = -0.5
Finally, substitute back in to the first equation to give 2 + G – 0.5 = 1. Thus, G = -0.5
Therefore, FGH = 2 x -0.5 x -0.5 = 0.5.

Question 18: D
The main artery to the lungs is the pulmonary artery, which gets blocked. The clot must therefore travel through the inferior vena cava and right side of the heart. It does not enter the superior vena cava or left (systemic) circulation.

Question 19: B
Note that the units are the same (M = moldm^{-3}), only the orders of magnitude are different. Convert the orders of magnitude to discover a 10^6 difference with more chloride than thyroxine

Question 20: E
This is a simple recall question. X rays have the shortest wavelength whilst microwaves have the longest wavelengths with visible light being somewhere in the middle. It is well worth your time remembering the basic positions of the components of the electromagnetic spectrum as it frequently gets tested in the BMAT.

Question 21: E
The way to solve this is to break the calculation down into parts, almost working backwards. The number of seconds in 66 weeks is given by:
= 60 x 60 x 24 x 7 x 66:
= (10 x 6) x (12 x 5) x (4 x 6) x 7 x (11 x 6)
= 1 x 4 x 5 x 6 x 6 x 6 x 7 x 10 x 11 x 12
= 1 x 4 x 5 x 6 x (6) x 7 x 10 x 11 x (12 x 6)
= 1 x 4 x 5 x 6 x (3 x 2) x 7 x 10 x 11 x (72)
= 1 x 2 x 3 x 4 x 5 x 6 x 7 x 10 x 11 x (9 x 8)
= 1 x 2 x 3 x 4 x 5 x 6 x 7 x 8 x 9 x 10 x11

Question 22: B
Glycogen is not a hormone, it is a polysaccharide storage product primarily found in muscle and the liver.

Question 23: C
The conceptual leap required for this question is that since the system is 100% efficient, energy won't be created or destroyed but merely transferred.
Thus, *Energy input into water = Gravitational potential energy at top of stream*
$100\ J\ per\ Second = mg\Delta h$
$h = \dfrac{100}{mg}$
$h = \dfrac{100}{1\ x\ 10} = 10\ m$

Question 24: D

Reflexes can be influenced by the brain e.g. if you willingly pick up a hot plate, you will be able to withstand much greater heat than if you touch it by accident and discover it is hot. Reflex actions are fast as they usually bypass the brain. Since they are mediated by nerves, they are much faster than endocrine responses. Most animals show basic reflexes like the heat-withdrawal reflex which requires both sensory and motor components.

Question 25: C

Remember the interior angles of a pentagon add up to 540° (three internal triangles), so each interior angle is 540/5 = 108°. Therefore angle **a** is 108°. Recalling that angles within a quadrilateral sum to 360°, we can calculate **b**. The larger angle in the central quadrilateral is 360° – 2 x 108° (angles at a point) = 144°. Therefore the remaining angle, **b** = (360 – 2(144)]/2 = 36°. The product of 36 and 108 is 3,888°.

Question 26: D

The key here is to note that the answers are several orders of magnitude apart so you can round the numbers to make your calculations easier:

Probability of bacteria being resistant to every antibiotic = P (Res to Antibiotic 1)x P (Res to Antibiotic 2)x P (Res to Antibiotic 3) x P (Res to Antibiotic 4)

$$= \frac{100}{10^{11}}x\frac{1000}{10^9}x\frac{100}{10^8}x\frac{1}{10^5}$$

$$= \frac{10^8}{10^{33}} = \frac{1}{10^{25}}$$

Question 27: F

All the above units are measures of power, the amount of work done per unit time.

END OF SECTION

Section 3

'The concept of medical euthanasia is dangerous and should never be permitted within the UK'

Explain the reasoning behind this statement. Suggest an argument against this statement. To what extent, should legislation regarding the prohibition of medical euthanasia in the UK be changed?

Euthanasia, from the Greek for *'mercy-killing'*, involves the active painless taking of patients' lives for those facing incurable physical, mental and social torment by disease. The practice is legal in certain parts of the world, including Switzerland, although the above statement argues that changes to the current law in the UK would have negative impact on the foundation of medical practice and welfare of doctors, patients and their families.

This is because the action of actively ending the life of patients may result in guilt-filled psychological effects on doctors. This is especially so as the profession in most cases aims to extend quantity of life.

In addition, the line between suffering patients who would and would not 'deserve' euthanasia is ambiguous. Some patients who have diseases that have a detrimental impact on their lives may opt for euthanasia, when actually there may be therapy or support to aid them in leading fulfilling lives. It would be also difficult to assess whether patients have the competence to judge their willingness for euthanasia, for example underlying depression that may be influencing their choice.

However, doctors should always have the quality of life of a patient at the forefront of treatment. In many debilitating disorders where patients require constant attention, physical support and lack fulfilling stimulation, the quality of life of patients is abysmal, for example in locked-in syndrome. For those who want to end their life, the relief of this suffering by the medical profession could be considered a caring act.

Moreover, euthanasia may relieve the burden of constant care faced by family members. Currently many patients make the journey to countries where medical euthanasia is legal, but as a result, family members face prosecution in good-willingly helping the patients to do so. Legalisation would relive the strain on family members of not only losing their patient relative but also of this criminal prospect.

However, in conclusion, the legislation should not be changed. Ultimately, it is too difficult to assess cases in which medical euthanasia would be acceptable. In addition, its legalisation may permit family members burdened with caring for a patient to pressurise patients into euthanasia. As a result, the effect of this concept revolving on 'mercy' towards a patient may end up being one of detriment.

'The obstruction of stem-cell research is directly responsible for death arising from stem-cell treatable diseases.'

Explain what this argument means. Argue the contrary. To what extend do you agree with the statement?

Stem-cell research offers the opportunity for a vast increase in our understanding of disease and generally of how the human body works. Being able to conduct research into the different areas that are involved in the growth of humans from sperm and egg and the formation of complex organisms will contribute greatly to our understanding not only of genetic and birth defects and their origin, but also to our understanding of disease. On top of that stem-cell research might theoretically offer the key to the cure of a variety of diseases such as spinal cord damage, organ failure or genetic defects. Being able to grow organs for transplantation for example provides a huge opportunity for the whole of mankind. Not having to wait for a needed organ will make the patient's life better and more bearable and also bring about a cure faster. Whilst the current status quo does allow some research into stem-cells, there are heavy restrictions when it comes to the use of human stem cells, not only because of the question at which point a baby becomes a human being.

Opposing the idea of deregulation of stem-cell research stands the main concern that all life is valuable and that includes the potential life represented by a foetus, the ultimate source of stem-cells used in research. The extraction of stem-cells for research is essentially nothing else as the destruction of potential human life, which is not acceptable. This concern is based on the idea that with the fusion of sperm and egg a new human being is being created that needs to be asked for consent in the participation of any research. As this is not possible for a foetus, some think that stem-cell research is unethical and in breach of the main principles underlying medical research and medical care in general. Another idea is that of 'the ends don't justify the means'. Whilst it is a reasonable prospect to expect that progress in stem-cell research will lead to the discovery of new treatment forms for a variety of severely impacting diseases, this does not justify the use of what essentially are non-consented human beings for research.

Stem-cell research most definitely holds a great deal of potential when it comes to the increase in medical knowledge. Being able to research into the area could potentially provide us with a greater understanding of a variety of biological processes as well with a cure to many forms of disease. None the less it is questionable if this alone justifies ignoring the fact that a foetus can potentially be killed by the extraction of stem cells which will directly cause the destruction of potentially healthy life. Ultimately there are arguments for and against stem-cell research. The majority hinge on the understanding of life as an untouchable unit. If we assume that a foetus only becomes a living human being after a certain period of time, this justifies research on the non-human state prior to that date. This is the commonly used legal interpretation of the issue facing researchers today.

'Imagination is more important than knowledge'

Albert Einstein

Explain how this statement could be interpreted in a medical setting. Argue to the contrary that knowledge is more important than imagination in medicine. To what extent do you agree with the statement?

Einstein alludes to creativity and imagination, rather than pure knowledge, being the driving force for scientific discovery. Medically, this could analogized as it being more important for doctors to be able to assimilate different thoughts and concepts together to come up with a differential diagnosis/ holistic management plan than it is to simply memorize all the underlying textbook theory.

On the contrary, unlike with many scientific discoveries, you cannot come up with a reliable and safe differential or management plan simply based on a hunch without a comprehensive underlying knowledge base.

If something goes wrong in scientific discovery, you can simply try again. With patients, this is not an option.

Guidelines and treatment recommendations e.g. from NICE/ specific medical bodies have largely removed the need for creativity in the management of patients. On the contrary, the gold standard is the practice of evidence-based medicine based on sound underlying knowledge.

It could be said that a strong knowledge base would help you diagnose/manage the most common conditions, while creativity and imagination help with the rarer conditions. Seeing as common is common, on average knowledge would be more important than imagination in treating most patients.

On balance, I believe that a strong knowledge base would make a good doctor, while a strong knowledge base together with imagination and creativity would make a great doctor. Knowledge can be seen as the core foundation needed by all doctors to practice safely and reliably. However the human body does not behave like a textbook and most conditions can present atypically. In this case, being able to integrate both these skills and use your underlying knowledge of pathophysiology to imagine how a condition may manifest atypically could be the key between spotting and missing a life-threatening diagnosis. E.g. An atypical presentation of Tuberculosis.

"The most important quality of a good doctor is a thorough understanding of science"

Explain what this statement means. Argue in favour of this statement. To what extent do you agree with it?

You should start the essay by showing your understanding of the question and pointing the reader in the direction you wish to take for the essay. Clarify any assumptions you will make.

The question talks about the most important quality of a good doctor – this implies that there are other important qualities of a good doctor, and it might help to identify what some of these are. It is not sufficient to simply argue that a thorough understanding of science is important – you must explain why it is more important than other important qualities.

Other qualities might include good communication skills, the ability to understand people's emotions, practical clinical skills, an understanding of how the healthcare system works and an understanding of your own limitations.

Address the reasons why a thorough understanding of science is important, then explain why these are more significant than the reasons supporting other important traits. Consider that the practice of medicine is based upon the scientific method, and all treatments to be funded by a modern healthcare system must be supported by evidence. Doctors need a thorough understanding of science in order to be able to work by these principles.

Note that science informs the correct treatment. Other skills might improve the benefit to patients, but without an appropriate treatment, informed by science, there will be no benefit.

A lack of knowledge or understanding of the science underlying medicine might lead to dangerous mistakes being made. This would go against the principle "first, do no harm" as first outlined in the Hippocratic Oath. In addition, patient safety is a fundamental and overarching principle of a safe and effective NHS.

State your position: to what extent do you agree with the statement and why. You might want to mitigate your support by reference to the importance of personal skills: better communication makes it more likely to find out what is wrong to inform the correct treatment, it makes it more likely the patient will understand and follow your suggested treatment regime, it might improve the placebo component of treatment (which is significant) and it might increase the patient's trust in you, leading to a better long-term relationship and thus benefiting their health.

Likewise with reference to practical skills, such as surgery, you might suggest that even if the right treatment is selected, without the right practical skills the treatment will not be beneficial to the patient and indeed could cause significant harm.

END OF PAPER

FINAL ADVICE

Arrive well rested, well fed and well hydrated

The BMAT is an intensive test, so make sure you're ready for it. Unlike the UKCAT, you'll have to sit this at a fixed time (normally at 9AM). Thus, ensure you get a good night's sleep before the exam (there is little point cramming) and don't miss breakfast. If you're taking water into the exam then make sure you've been to the toilet before so you don't have to leave during the exam. Make sure you're well rested and fed in order to be at your best!

Move on

If you're struggling, move on. Every question has equal weighting and there is no negative marking. In the time it takes to answer on hard question, you could gain three times the marks by answering the easier ones. Be smart to score points- especially in section two where some questions are far easier than others.

Make Notes on your Essay

Some universities may ask you questions on your BMAT essay at the interview. Sometimes you may have the interview as late as March which means that you **MUST** make short notes on the essay title and your main arguments after the essay. This is especially important if you're applying to UCL and Cambridge where the essay is discussed more frequently.

Afterword

Remember that the route to a high score is your approach and practice. Don't fall into the trap that *"you can't prepare for the BMAT"*– this could not be further from the truth. With knowledge of the test, some useful time-saving techniques and plenty of practice you can dramatically boost your score.

Work hard, never give up and do yourself justice.

Good Luck!

Acknowledgements

I would like to thank Rohan and the UniAdmissions Tutors for all their hard work and advice in compiling this book, and both my parents and Meg for their continued unwavering support.

Matthew

About UniAdmissions

UniAdmissions is an educational consultancy that specialises in supporting **applications to Medical School and to Oxbridge**.

Every year, we work with hundreds of applicants and schools across the UK. From free resources to our *Ultimate Guide Books* and from intensive courses to bespoke individual tuition – with a team of **300 Expert Tutors** and a proven track record, it's easy to see why UniAdmissions is the **UK's number one admissions company**.

To find out more about our support like intensive **BMAT courses** and **BMAT tuition** check out www.uniadmissions.co.uk/bmat

Your Free Book

Thanks for purchasing this Ultimate Guide Book. Readers like you have the power to make or break a book – hopefully you found this one useful and informative. If you have time, *UniAdmissions* would love to hear about your experiences with this book.

As thanks for your time we'll send you another ebook from our Ultimate Guide series absolutely <u>FREE</u>!

How to Redeem Your Free Ebook in 3 Easy Steps

1) Either scan the QR code or find the book you have on your Amazon purchase history or email your receipt to help find the book on Amazon.

2) On the product page at the Customer Reviews area, click on 'Write a customer review.' Write your review and post it! Copy the review page or take a screen shot of the review you have left.

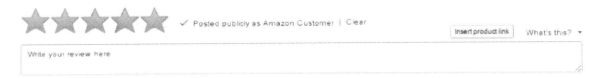

1) Head over to www.uniadmissions.co.uk/free-book and select your chosen free ebook! You can choose from:

✓ BMAT Mock Papers
✓ BMAT Past Paper Solutions
✓ The Ultimate Oxbridge Interview Guide
✓ The Ultimate UCAS Personal Statement Guide
✓ The Ultimate BMAT Guide – 800 Practice Questions

Your ebook will then be emailed to you – it's as simple as that!
Alternatively, you can buy all the above titles at

www.uniadmissions.co.uk/our-books

BMAT Online Course

If you're looking to improve your BMAT score in a short space of time, our **BMAT Online Course** is perfect for you. The BMAT Online Course offers all the content of a traditional course in a single easy-to-use online package-available instantly after checkout. The online videos are just like the classroom course, ready to watch and re-watch at home or on the go and all with our expert Oxbridge tuition and advice.

You'll get full access to all of our BMAT resources including:

✓ Copy of our acclaimed book "The Ultimate BMAT Guide"
✓ Full access to extensive BMAT online resources including:
✓ 10 hours of BMAT on-demand lectures
✓ 8 complete mock papers
✓ 800 practice questions
✓ Fully worked solutions for all BMAT past papers since 2003
✓ Ongoing Tutor Support until Test date – never be alone again.

The course is normally £99 but you can get **£ 20 off** by using the code *"UAONLINE20"* at checkout.

https://www.uniadmissions.co.uk/product/bmat-online-course/

£20 VOUCHER:

UAONLINE20

Medical Interview Online Course

If you've got an upcoming interview for medical school but unable to attend our intensive interview course– this is the perfect **Medical Interview Online Course** for you. The Online Course has:

✓ 40 medical interview on-demand videos covering Oxbridge and MMI-style questions.
✓ Copy of the book "The Ultimate Medical Interview Guide."
✓ Over 150 past interview questions and answers.
✓ Ongoing Tutor Support until your interview – never be alone again

The online course is normally £99 but you can get £20 off by using the code *"UAONLINE20"* at checkout.

https://www.uniadmissions.co.uk/product/online-medical-interview-course/

£20 VOUCHER:
UAONLINE20

UKCAT Online Course

If you're looking to improve your UKCAT score in a short space of time, our **UKCAT Online Course** is perfect for you. The UKCAT Online Course offers all the content of a traditional course in a single easy-to-use online package-available instantly after checkout. The online videos are just like the classroom course, ready to watch and re-watch at home or on the go and all with our expert Oxbridge tuition and advice.

You'll get full access to all of our UKCAT resources including:

- ✓ Copy of our acclaimed book "The Ultimate UKCAT Guide"
- ✓ Full access to extensive UKCAT online resources including:
- ✓ 10 hours of UKCAT on-demand lectures
- ✓ 6 complete mock papers
- ✓ 1250 practice questions
- ✓ Fully worked solutions for all UKCAT past papers since 2003
- ✓ Ongoing Tutor Support until Test date – never be alone again.

The course is normally £99 but you can get **£ 20 off** by using the code *"UAONLINE20"* at checkout.

https://www.uniadmissions.co.uk/product/ukcat-online-course/

£20 VOUCHER:
UAONLINE20

Printed in Great
Britain
by Amazon